The Light Between the Leaves

Also by Scott Eilers, PsyD, LP

For When Everything Is Burning

The Light Between the Leaves

6 TRUTHS YOUR THERAPIST WON'T TELL YOU ABOUT HEALING DEPRESSION AND TRAUMA

Scott Eilers, PsyD, LP

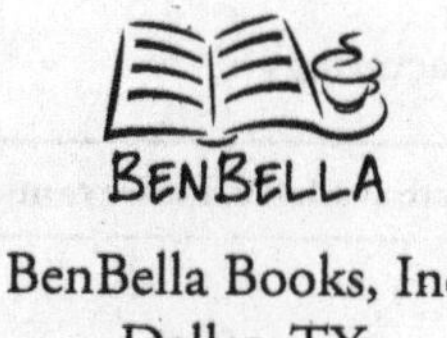

BenBella Books, Inc.
Dallas, TX

BenBella Books, Inc.
8080 N. Central Expressway
Suite 1700
Dallas, TX 75206
benbellabooks.com
Send feedback to feedback@benbellabooks.com

BenBella is a federally registered trademark.

Printed in the United States of America
10 9 8 7 6 5 4 3 2 1

Library of Congress Control Number: 2025040043
ISBN 9781637748282 (trade paperback)
ISBN 9781637748299 (electronic)

Editing by Claire Schulz and Sarah Modlin
Copyediting by Scott Calamar
Proofreading by Ashley Casteel and Martha Gallant
Text design and composition by PerfecType, Nashville, TN
Cover design by Morgan Carr
Printed by Lake Book Manufacturing

This work is dedicated to all who know the pain of having their harshest critic, biggest detractor, and true nemesis living inside of themselves. I know your fight, and you are not alone in it. I see you and you inspire me every day.

If these words resonate and you'd like to stay connected, the code below will take you to more resources I created for you.

Contents

Introduction (Born Broken) 1

TRUTH ONE: BEGIN WITHIN

The Story (The Road) 21

The Lesson (Isolation) 28

The Application (How to Care for Yourself) 35

TRUTH TWO: ENVY IS IGNORANCE

The Story (The Lake) 49

The Lesson (Nemesis) 56

The Application (Celebrate, Identify, Locate, Pursue) 64

TRUTH THREE: DON'T LET THE DARKNESS IN

The Story (The Forest) 79

The Lesson (Regrowth) 86

The Application (Scrutinize the Lies) 95

TRUTH FOUR: PULL THE WEEDS

The Story (The Flowers) 107
The Lesson (Invasive Species) 113
The Application (Managing Your Ecosystem) 123

TRUTH FIVE: LOVE WHAT YOU HAVE

The Story (The Farm) 137
The Lesson (Lost Forever) 143
The Application (Remember What Matters Most) 150

TRUTH SIX: KEEP THE WATER FLOWING

The Story (The River) 163
The Lesson (Stuck in the Mud) 169
The Application (Never Stagnate) 175

Conclusion (Patterns) 185
Acknowledgments 195

Introduction

Born Broken

I was awake before the sun, but I wasn't the first. My son's smiling face and the mewing of his kitten greeted me when I reached the main floor. A thin, fresh layer of snow blanketed the expanse of grassland and forest visible from our living room window, but the creek dividing our property was running strong, unbothered by the low temperatures of winter in the Midwest. I watched the water flow for a moment and took note of the peace I felt within. Something about moving water has always calmed me. With a quick turn of a key and the flick of a lighter, a gentle and inviting glow from our gas fireplace warmed the room.

"Daddy, want to play Roblox?"

"You know it!"

Thirty minutes later we were joined by my just-awoken wife and daughter. Within minutes, our home smelled of bacon and coffee. Plans were made for the day: grocery store and recycling center in the morning, sanding and painting trim in our fun fixer-upper project home midday, and maybe some ice fishing with my brother in the evening. The following day we planned to enjoy some time with extended family, make a run to the hardware store for a few more home improvement projects, and cap off the weekend with pizza and board games, just the four of us.

Sometimes I remember to appreciate moments like these, but not always. Weekends like the one I just described aren't noteworthy for me at this point in my life. I have a career that I love, a consistent place to live, and I'm part of a warm, loving family. And that, in and of itself, is special. That I can experience peace, connection, excitement, accomplishment, and joy on an average weekend of my life is nothing short of a miracle. I spent much of my life thoroughly convinced I would have none of these things.

In fact, it really wasn't that long ago that I didn't care if I lived or died.

Life Isn't Always Beautiful

For years, I had only one desire. I just wanted my pain to stop, and I could only imagine one way out. I asked for it in my mind, and sometimes out loud.

End me.

Stop wasting my time.

Do it before I do it myself, because I'm getting tired of waiting.

It's not like I had anything to look forward to. Every day was exactly the same:

Open my eyes.

Curse.

Drag my unwilling body out of bed.

Search desperately for my little escapes from my own life: listening to the saddest, angriest music imaginable because it makes me feel a little less alone; talking to the one or two people I don't find insufferable; taking a warm bath when it's all over and feeling the pain of the day wash away in the water, even if only for a moment.

My existence was a void draining the lives of those closest to me. Nothing filled the emptiness, like someone forgot to put my soul inside of my body. Companions were short-lived; nobody wants to spend too much time around someone like me, lest some of the brokenness rub off on them. I was aimless, alone, and miserable.

I never felt completely hopeless in the literal "there is no chance this ever gets better" sense. I believed with my whole heart that there was something out there for me, some just-right combination of people, places, and things that could bring me lasting joy. I also believed with my whole heart that I would never find these things. I felt like a prisoner inside my own mind. No matter where I went and what I did, I couldn't escape the torture that was being myself. Every day was punishment, a ceaseless penance with no end in sight.

And it was all my fault.

But It Can Be

I've been the same person in all chapters of my story, including the two you've just read about. The capability to be both individuals, and anything in between them, has always existed within me. That's not because I'm special in any way; we're all capable of unbelievable change. Even if you feel more like the lost, tormented version of myself, it's not too bad for you to build a life that feels meaningful and fulfilling most of the time. There's absolutely nothing I've done that you can't do. You might be skeptical, but I'm sure of it.

There's something inside of you that you've only seen glimpses of. Fleeting feelings that never seem to last, even though you so desperately want them to. Hints and visions of a person you can't quite believe you could ever become. I know you see them sometimes, even if only for a second. Maybe it feels terrifying to hold on to that feeling for any real length of time, like the crash from the emotional high of thinking you're not utterly devoid of value and hope could literally kill you. It's much safer to stay at the bottom, where no unexpected falls can happen because you cannot possibly sink any lower. But I want you to know that this other person still exists within you, and as long as you continue to breathe, they will never die.

It's possible to find that person deep within yourself and drag them out of you. Even if it has been decades since that version of yourself was at the forefront of your being, or even if it never has been. Even if it has never left the tiny, protected pocket inside of you where it resides. Eventually, what you first wear as a mask can become your true face. It can become your genuine way of being in this world rather than a tool to placate others who otherwise will ask too many uncomfortable questions that they haven't earned the answers to. I know how terrifying it is to even think of putting a raw, authentic, vulnerable version of yourself out there into this savage, callous world we live in, but it can change absolutely everything.

No matter what you achieve in life, you will never receive anything more precious than what you already have. You were born with an invaluable treasure, something wonderful and fragile, and something that can never be taken from you.

That treasure is you.

I know how this may sound. In your head, alarm bells are ringing, red flags being raised. These are bold claims, and bold claims usually come from people who are working some angle. You know the type. People who talk a big game about how great you are and how awesome your life could be but can't back up their empty assertions with any real concepts or strategies. You may feel a slight boost in your mood when you read their generic reassurances, but once you get past those and the rush wears off, nothing of substance remains. You feel just as hollow and empty as before, but now you're angry that another person raised your hopes before proving to you, yet again, that they cannot help you.

I promise you I'm just as sick of those people as you are. As a licensed clinical psychologist and a practicing psychotherapist, I spend quite a bit of time trying to deprogram people from the toxic positivity and oversimplified messages causing them to endlessly shame themselves for not feeling happy enough. We're told that everything happens for an acceptable, understandable reason, which means we're being asked to believe that genocide, mass shootings, sex trafficking, children dying, and chronic mental illness all serve some greater good. We're slapped with labels like "pessimist," "negative," or even "treatment resistant" for making the mistake of questioning whether the world we live in is actually supposed to feel good—and asserting that if it is, our tendencies must not have been considered when it was being designed.

So no, I'm not that kind of person, and this is not going to be that kind of book. Many of the cults have left their compounds and moved on to Instagram and TikTok, and it absolutely terrifies me. Science, logic, and reasoning are my safe spaces. I despise placations and empty promises. People who oversimplify the immensely complex and arduous journey of life that we're all on make me want to vomit in irritation. I'm pretty sure that's biologically possible. But even within the context of my absolute disgust at peddlers of false hope, I still stand by my earlier statement about how important and incredible you are, and I will never back down from it.

Because you're a freaking incredible creature, and it would be scientifically ignorant to say otherwise.

If you could magnify the inner architecture of your brain by one thousand times and walk around inside of it, you would see something more intricate than the Sistine Chapel, more beautiful than the *Moonlight Sonata*, and more complex than the Milky Way (the galaxy, not the candy bar . . . well, actually both). It would be the most jaw-dropping, awe-inspiring experience of your life. You spend every day inside this miracle of creation, failing to appreciate how absolutely incredible it is.

In your possession are roughly one hundred billion brain cells, also called neurons. Each neuron has between one thousand and ten thousand connections to other neurons, making for approximately one hundred trillion possible neural connections inside of you. Every change in neural connectivity modifies you ever so slightly. When two neurons communicate for the first time, something new is created inside of you. When two neurons that used to communicate stop doing so, a belief that once felt solid and inarguable is left behind. Your mind is constantly shedding its previous skin. Connections grow, and connections die; associations are formed and lost. The structure and functioning of your brain change every second of every day. The mind that you possess when you finish reading this sentence will be slightly different than the one you possessed when you started reading it: Each modification makes a new you. Individually, none of these changes are immense. But hundreds of thousands of changes over a long enough period of time? That can change you from someone who resents their own existence into someone who enthusiastically embraces their life every day.

And we haven't covered the best part yet. The real highlight here is that this unbelievable treasure isn't just some abstract part of nature for you to observe. All of this belongs to you; and you, more than any other person, are in charge of how it grows and develops. You get to build your own little world inside of yourself. Reshaping and remaking your brain is your life's greatest work: You are an artist, an architect, and an engineer.

Everything you've witnessed and experienced in your life—every technological advancement, every marvelous sunset, every intricate ecosystem—isn't even close in scale to the complexity of what lives inside of you. Your inner world is incomprehensibly vast and unbelievably intricate. The next time you look up in wonder at the stars in a cloudless night sky, remember that you have something even more beautiful and immense within yourself.

I know it doesn't always feel that way. Life is a gift for all, but not all gifts are equally thoughtful. Sometimes the gift of life feels personal, relevant, and carefully created. Sometimes it feels more like a homemade clown sweater, presented with a crooked smile and a sinister, obligatory statement about love and appreciation. But no matter where you began your journey, and no matter what the people who created you had in mind for you (if they had anything in mind at all), you get to decide where to go from here. After all, you weren't a consenting adult in the matter of your own creation, and nobody can stop you from disobeying a contract you never signed.

I Wasn't Meant for This World

Some people appear to be naturally happy and content unless there's something happening in their lives to cause them distress, while others of us are naturally unhappy and discontented unless there's something happening in our lives to actively create a positive emotional experience. I am the second type of person. There is next to no natural happiness, lightness, or joy within me. I must earn every ounce of it, and that's the way I've always been.

For most of my life, I would have told you that I wasn't made for this world. I've always seemed to have a special ability to find extreme misery in the things that are meant to make me happy. It's sort of like the world's worst superpower. Things that are supposed to be calming to me often stress me out. Activities that are meant to be fun and enjoyable sometimes throw me into existential despair. I don't do it on purpose. I didn't set out to be this way, and in fact I would very much prefer not to be.

Peace, joy, and contentment are not my default emotional states when nothing is majorly wrong, and for most of my life they've been rare and fleeting experiences requiring some incomprehensibly precise alignment of external stimuli, internal mindset, and emotional state. I spent half my life chasing these magical moments, trying desperately to re-experience them through a mix of people, substances, and dissociation. At one point, I thought nothing short of a brain transplant could fix me—I was just born broken.

My baby milestones book legitimately reads like a supervillain origin story. Highlights include:

- Three months old: "Smiling babies seem to make him cry."
- Six months old: "He really doesn't seem to want to sleep at night . . ."
- One year old: "He only eats tuna, peas, and ice cream cones." (My addition: This doesn't mean "ice cream cones containing ice cream." Literally just the cones. And how did I not die of mercury poisoning from all that tuna?)

Somehow, I managed not to traumatize them into making me an only child, which is a minor miracle in and of itself. They decided to have two more children, probably hoping I was some type of anomaly and the others would be normal. (Spoiler alert: We're all total weirdos in different ways.) I can't imagine what it must have been like to raise me. I've always wondered if they secretly questioned whether their biological child had been abducted and replaced with an alien baby gathering data on humanity for purposes of future world domination.

If you're wondering if things got better when puberty started, picture me laughing maniacally right now. If you don't know what I look like, just picture Tom Cruise laughing maniacally right now. I don't particularly resemble Tom Cruise; I just find it really easy to picture him laughing maniacally. Things got so, so much worse during my adolescence. I started to realize that not everyone thought and felt like me. This caused me to spend a lot of time pondering exactly who and what I was, where I was supposed to be, and how my horrible mistake of a life came to be.

I developed metacognition (the ability to think about my own thoughts) and shortly thereafter realized that I absolutely should not be allowed to have metacognition. I hated my own mind so much I fantasized about defragmenting it like a computer hard drive, rearranging all my neurons in a more functional alignment that didn't make me despise everyone and everything. Including myself. I tried desperately to find other people who thought and felt like I did, which resulted in the assembly of one of the oddest peer groups ever created. We were sort of like the depression Avengers.

Looking back on those experiences today feels a lot like waking up from a vague, confusing nightmare; you remember that it was awful, but you can't really put together all the pieces to explain exactly what happened. You can't quite rationalize the sick feeling in the pit of your stomach that won't go away and gnaws at your mind. I remember feeling like I was living inside of a void. It was like a personal black hole followed me wherever I went. Other people could see it, or at least sense it, and they kept their distance from me for fear of falling in.

I felt almost no joy, no motivation, no excitement. It was emotional poverty. Every day was a war of attrition, any thoughts of thriving or enjoying myself were long forgotten. My only question was whether the shallow reserves of energy and focus I possessed would be enough to fulfill the bare minimum of the academic, social, and physical demands placed upon me. Most days the answer was a deafening "no" that echoed in the sprawling, vacant warehouse of my mind.

Although I would have told you then that the problem was everyone except me, I understand now that I was unintentionally making all the wrong choices every day. My attempts at digging myself out of this hole were functionally equivalent to someone flailing wildly after falling through thin ice on a frozen lake. (If you happen to be unfamiliar with frozen lake safety, this is the thing you are definitely not supposed to do and which will likely kill you. I promise to thoroughly explain any and every outdoorsy Midwest metaphor, of which there will be many.) Purposely withholding my best effort from every endeavor so I had a reasonable excuse when I failed. Acting out in ways that drove everyone away, so I had a reasonable excuse when nobody liked me. Refusing to take even the slightest, simplest action that might have helped me improve my situation.

That's why I believe it was my fault. I didn't make myself this way, but the only person with the power to change me was me. And I was going about it in all the wrong ways.

But I Can Create a World That Works for Me

Like so many who work in mental health, my interest in this field came first and foremost from a desire to help myself. I reasoned that, if there was an entire field of study dedicated to understanding and improving the functioning of the human brain, surely I could figure out what the heck was wrong with me and what exactly I should do about it. And so, I made that the focus of my education.

I'm going to summarize that ten-year chapter of my life with a single sentence: I did not find the answers I was seeking.

Every concept, every study, and every therapeutic technique I learned about seemed to be based on the same faulty principle; the idea that, underneath the problems, the symptoms, and the struggles lies a naturally happy person whose existence is being repressed by painful or disappointing childhood events. This has never been my truth.

I was unhappy before anything was "wrong." My inner child has oppositional-defiant disorder; he doesn't even listen to my outer adult. Trying to give my authentic self a voice would resemble the scene from *The Ring* where Rachel recovers Samara's body from the well: brief hope followed by utter chaos. The thoughts and feelings that run below the surface in my mind, even today, are not those of a man with a heart of gold underneath a hard exterior. There is, and always has been, an inexplicable darkness within me. I did not ask for it and I do not like it, but it remains.

I've had a pretty good life, objectively speaking. You might think that someone like me experienced some horrific trauma early on to create this darkness inside of me. I'd love to tell you that was the case, because I think it would make a lot more sense than the truth, which is that I've always been this way for no apparent reason. I used to invent stories of horrible things I'd experienced because it seemed like the only way my emotions could ever make sense to anyone was if they were paired with a tragic backstory. Absolutely nothing happened to me to make me this way; I was born like this. Born dissatisfied. Born angry. Born discontent. Born broken.

I can't just wake up and experience happiness. I'm not doing anything to sabotage it or suppress it; happiness doesn't know where I live. I have to pursue it with every fiber of my being, stalking it like a lion stalks a wounded gazelle, because it will never find me on its own. Left to its own devices, my brain does not work the way I want it to. It isn't naturally my friend, and it doesn't inherently want to help me. I've had to tirelessly, relentlessly train it to behave the way I want it to.

When I didn't find my answers in therapy, in graduate school, or from other people with similar experiences, I decided to seek them elsewhere. There was one phase of my life where I could recall being truly, deeply happy despite the war constantly raging inside of me: During the brief period of my childhood when I lived in a little cabin in the woods with my family, the war seemed to quiet down. There was something about that place that changed me. I thought differently, I felt differently, and I lived differently when I was there. As an adult, I knew my lifestyle was different, and that things could never be exactly as they were back then, but I wondered what would happen if I tried to make my life as similar as possible to that time. If it worked once, maybe it could work again.

The most important lessons I've learned didn't come from classes or jobs, supervisors or mentors. They didn't come from books, or social media, or therapy. They came from somewhere far less academic and far more primitive. They came from the woods and the rivers and the lakes of my childhood. They came from calmly, patiently observing my inner experience; from trying to figure out what was going on in there and how I could change it. There have been so many moments in my life when I was observing something seemingly unimportant or miniscule, only to realize I was seeing something much greater: a truth, principle, or pattern that determines every facet of my life.

There is an entire world inside of you. A vast ecosystem full of interconnected parts. Sometimes these parts work together harmoniously, but they can easily become unbalanced and dysfunctional.

You're the manager of this inner world. Whether it thrives and flourishes or rots and decays is entirely dictated by your choices.

I want to teach you how to take care of that world. Nourishing your inner ecosystem and helping it thrive is not common sense. It often involves doing the exact opposite of what is considered culturally normal.

Let me make something very clear before we go any further: What I'm going to be encouraging you to do will be incredibly difficult. The changes I made to get from where I used to be to where I am today were anything but minor. What I'm offering you in these pages is not a series of little tweaks or adjustments to make to your life. It's more like a prairie fire, a controlled burn of your mind to flush away all the dead and decaying matter that prevents new growth from flourishing. I had to relearn how to live, and most of my beliefs and behaviors did not survive the process.

I also want to clarify that I am by no means against people being in therapy. Just because I didn't find what I was looking for there doesn't mean nobody will. And providing therapy, particularly for people with potentially disabling conditions such as bipolar disorder, severe depression, severe anxiety, post-traumatic stress disorder, borderline personality disorder, anorexia, and bulimia, is still a huge part of my career. If I come across as negative or pessimistic towards my chosen profession, it's just because I've personally been let down by it during my times of greatest need, and there is some resentment there, not because I think it's a worthless service that doesn't help anybody.

My battle is by no means over. I still feel the pull of a depressive spiral at times, but I can almost always step around it. I still feel the spark of misery inside of me on occasion, but I know how to extinguish it before it reignites into the raging bonfire that once consumed everything in my life. My darkest periods now last for minutes, hours, or, on very rare occasions, days. Weeks, months, or even years of despair are a thing of the past. I am winning. Against all odds, despite being born with an utterly disenchanted and nihilistic worldview, I've managed to build a life that feels very, very good to me most of the time.

And I'm going to teach you the most important conclusions from my experience in six stories and lessons.

How This Book Works

Each of these six chapters consists of three sections:

The Story: A summary of the initial experience that demonstrated a critical life principle to me. I believe that, just as in therapy, understanding the backstory to a concept is critical for fully comprehending it and being able to apply it to your own life. There have been so many times in my own journey where I couldn't, or wouldn't, use a skill or a technique that I technically understood until I knew more about where it came from and why it worked. That's why I start each chapter with a little bit of personal history.

The Lesson: What I learned from the experience described in the story. Each of these six experiences had a meaning far beyond what happened in the initial moment. My observations of principles demonstrated in the natural world contained priceless truths that I never found in classrooms or therapy offices.

The Application: Practical techniques for using the concept described in "The Lesson" in your own life. I don't want to teach you something important and then leave you to figure out what to do with that information. I'm going to spell out, in as much detail as possible, exactly how you can integrate these critical lessons into your daily functioning.

Of course, how you use this book is entirely up to you. If you aren't interested in the backstory and just want to get straight to the part where I give you ideas on how to get better, feel free to skip right to the application section. I'm not the book police.

I sincerely hope that you can learn from my experiences, but more than anything, I just hope that upon reading a bit more about my background, you feel less alone in this world. I grew up thinking I was the only person who thought and felt the way that I did. It's clear to me now that this wasn't the case, and learning that earlier in life would have saved me a tremendous amount of heartache. Hopefully these six truths can transform your life the way they transformed mine.

Truth One

Begin Within

The Story

The Road

I spent much of my childhood in a cabin on the shores of the most beautiful lake imaginable. Twelve hundred immaculate acres of pure, clean water hidden away inside of a massive national forest. Our lake was known for being one of the clearest in the county. It was so deep and blue it looked almost oceanic. No matter how many times I saw it, it never failed to take my breath away. It was also incredibly full of, and surrounded by, vibrant life in so many forms.

Every species of fish had a distinct personality. Gentle and curious sunfish roamed the shallows, watching us swim and eating bread from our hands. Bass stayed farther back, lurking cautiously within the weeds and under lily pads. Yellow perch schooled sporadically across the lake, seemingly found almost anywhere you could be bothered to look for them. My little brother once caught one in the absolute middle of the lake while we were boating at a high rate of speed. He swears to this day that it's a clear indicator of his superior fishing skill, but I maintain that it reflects much more on the decision-making capabilities of that particular perch. Black crappie, our favorite fish to eat, stayed mostly hidden during the day, emerging at dusk to feed on bugs and minnows. You could find them by spotting the gentle ripples created as they snatched insects from the surface, breaking the unblemished glass of the water.

Further out into the depths, northern pike and muskellunge would hunt for anything they could fit into their toothy jaws. Schools of walleye hugged the bottom, rarely seen unless you knew exactly where to find them. We would regularly come across schools of thousands of ciscoes, oblivious baitfish that crucially maintain the health of the food chain. Sometimes we would even encounter a prehistoric bowfin, an odd creature that looks like an eel/fish hybrid with the face of a brontosaurus. Whitefish burrowed down fifty feet or more into the water column, occasionally rising to the surface at night. Every now and then we'd catch glimpses of fish we couldn't immediately identify, furthering our sense of mystery and wonder at what lay just beyond the reaches of our sight.

There were a few houses and resorts on the lake, but most of it was bordered with every type of beautiful northern tree imaginable. Pine. Fir. Oak. Birch. Alder. Cedar. Juniper. Each releasing a subtly distinct scent when its branches were thrown onto a campfire. The horizon in every direction was brown and green blending into blue and white. The white pines stretched impossibly far into the sky, and we constantly searched for the biggest ones we could find; they were our rural versions of skyscrapers.

Birds of all kinds called the lake home. Small songbirds littered the forest, and the hammering of woodpeckers, including the massive and endangered pileated, was a near-constant soundtrack. Ducks, loons, geese, and occasionally even swans roamed across the surface of the lake looking for food and nesting ground. Bald eagles and ospreys prowled the sky, catching fish even when we could find none and building massive nests overlooking the water. Herons roamed the shallows, waiting with statuesque patience to pick off hapless bait-fish. My brother was even once attacked by a bittern, an odd creature that resembles an elongated kiwi with a beak and legs, which was described in our bird book as "a shy, reclusive bird that avoids human contact at all costs."

The surrounding forests remained mostly as they were hundreds of years ago, generally unseen and untouched by humankind. You could see a few feet into it, at most, before your line of sight was blocked by thousands of overlapping trunks and branches. Deer were a near-daily sighting, especially in the middle of summer when the does introduced their fawns to the rest of the world. Raccoons, opossums, fishers, and martins would emerge from the dense forest nightly, especially after we'd spent the evening cleaning fish in the yard, to scavenge for leftovers. On occasion, we would even have startling and brief encounters with bears and wolves.

I spent all summer playing, exploring, and adventuring along with my little sister and brother, respectively two and four years younger than me. We'd glide back and forth on a zip line built between two poles that were once used for drying clothes. We'd swim in the lake, playing with float toys and looking for unique treasures to immortalize on the shelf adorning our bedroom wall. We fished nearly every day, weather permitting. Sometimes we would even defy the weather and fish in a rainstorm, often with fantastic results. We played volleyball in the side yard, on a comically lopsided net strung between two birch trees. We searched our yard for unique bugs, leaves, sticks, and rocks. Many nights we'd build a bonfire on the shore of the lake and roast marshmallows, and occasionally spiders (we didn't eat the spiders, though).

Ours was the fourth-to-last house on Birch Lake Trail, a winding, twisting gravel road about a mile long. For the longest time I didn't realize we even had a street name or a house number. There were no mailboxes and basically no utilities or services of any kind beyond electricity. We had baseboard heating and no air conditioning. Our television was only used to watch the few movies we owned on VHS; the lone channel that came in through the antenna rarely had anything of interest. We had to bag up our own garbage and take it to the dump every week.

There was nothing on our little road but more houses. Some of these houses had people living in them year-round, but many were vacation homes and spent most of the year empty. The little ditches on either side of the road would fill with water and algae after the spring rains. Frogs moved in during the summer, with tadpoles soon to follow. We'd catch the frogs with dry flies, nets, or even our bare hands. We found treasures on every outing: abandoned turtle shells, unique rocks, beautiful wildflowers, and interesting bugs to catch and put in our bug boxes.

Birch Lake Trail sits on a peninsula between two bays of the lake. It's surrounded by water on both sides and dead-ends into the driveway of the last house on the road, meaning there's only one way in and out. At the entrance, connecting the gravel road to a small, paved two-lane highway, was a general store. It served the role of gas station, grocery store, bait shop, gift shop, and later, real estate office, all at once. That road was the only access point to our house other than our dock on the lake, a single swath of gravel carved through the dense forest. The only thing connecting us to the rest of the world.

Besides the general store on the corner of our road and the highway itself, there wasn't much of interest anywhere near our home. The closest little town was an unincorporated community with a population of about one hundred. It had a tiny antique store, a laundromat with a diner attached to it, a small logging company, an RV campground, and a bar and grill with a hotel that nobody ever stayed in. That was pretty much it. Everything else around us was either trees or water. It was a wild, natural, mostly uncivilized area.

We could, and often did, walk to the general store. It was only about a mile from our house. However, if we needed anything beyond what we could purchase at the general store, we had to travel ten miles north to a town of about five hundred, or thirty miles south to a city of about twelve thousand. We went to the city weekly for groceries and other necessities. Occasionally we would have visitors over or attend events in one of the neighboring towns, but on many days, we didn't have any human contact other than with one another.

If this sounds like paradise to you, it usually felt that way to me, too. It was, and still is, my favorite place in the world. I revisit it regularly, each time thinking my memories of it might be exaggerated by nostalgia, only to be proven wrong; it never fails to fill me with the same wonder I experienced as a child. The natural beauty and the scope of adventures one could experience in that region are unimaginable; I worked very hard to paint a picture of it for you through my words, yet these paragraphs do no justice to what it was like living there. My memories of my time in that place with my family are precious treasures that I would not trade for any amount of riches, fame, or talent. But there was one massive drawback to living there: an immense shortcoming that, under certain circumstances, made our little secluded paradise feel more like a deserted island

It was that our only connection to the rest of the world was a short, barely maintained, gravel road. Our ability to access people, resources, and experiences beyond those found in our backyard was completely dependent upon the existence of this little trail. If anything happened to it, we would be fully cut off from the rest of the world.

I wasn't consciously aware that we were constantly living on the verge of complete isolation, but I remember the exact moment when I first realized it. I was ten years old, and my sister and I decided that we needed some extra spending money for a couple of new water toys we had seen at the general store. We gathered up some fishing lures we didn't use anymore, "treasures" (like old turtle shells and wasp nests), and a few older toys, and carried a folding card table down to the end of our driveway to have a "garage sale." I vaguely remember our parents telling us that our idea probably wasn't going to work, but I didn't understand why. We sat at the bottom of that driveway for hours in the sweltering midsummer heat, and a total of two cars drove by. We made precisely zero dollars in sales.

Garage sales don't work very well when you live close to the end of a dead-end road. That day served as a stark reminder of the isolation of our living situation and the crisis that would instantly befall us if our road were to become blocked.

And every now and then the road *would* be blocked. Limbs or even trees could fall across it during a windstorm, and some of them were too heavy to move by hand and too large to drive over. In the winter, the snow could get so deep that the road couldn't be used until it was plowed. Sometimes the heavy spring or summer rains would create so much mud that even a vehicle with four-wheel drive couldn't find traction. On days like these we truly were trapped at home with one another, locked up and isolated until the road was cleared, and we could rejoin the rest of the world. Everything else was still out there just like it was before, but we had no way to access it. We couldn't reach the grocery store to restock our refrigerator. We couldn't reach the hospital should we need medical care. We couldn't get to the gas station to refuel our vehicles. Our lives were essentially on hold until the road was fixed.

I learned so many important lessons while living on Birch Lake Trail. How to catch, clean, and cook fish. How to tie knots. How to build a campfire. How to set minnow traps. How to drive a boat. How to unhook a fish. Even, unfortunately, how to unhook a person. But the lesson that meant the most to me wasn't a skill that could be taught. It was a fundamental truth about life that I live by every day:

When there's a single pathway connecting you to the rest of the world, you need to take care of that pathway as if your life depends on it. Because it literally does.

The Lesson

Isolation

When my first depressive episode hit, there was something in the core of it that felt familiar. It was a feeling I remember from my childhood, even if for a completely different reason: the sensation of everything good in this world suddenly seeming very far away and completely inaccessible to me. I knew that there was still love, joy, and peace somewhere out there in the world, but I couldn't seem to reach them. It felt like they were galaxies away from me, with no traversable path between where I was and where I longed to be.

There are many ways we can become trapped and isolated, and they don't all involve logs, snow, or mud. We can also become trapped within ourselves, because every last one of us lives on a psychological dead-end dirt road with only one way in and one way out. Having experienced both the literal disconnection of Birch Lake Trail being blocked, and the emotional disconnection of feeling completely cut off from the world and everyone and everything in it, I can say this with confidence: The latter is far worse.

The road connecting you to the rest of the world is the functioning of your mind (specifically your prefrontal cortex, but I'll save the neuroscience lesson for the next section). Have you ever had the feeling of being alone in a crowd of people, or of doing something that "should" be fun, but instead feeling bored, sad, or empty? The feelings that were missing from those moments, the sense of connection to those around you or the ability to enjoy a generally pleasant experience, got stuck on the road of your mind, and they didn't make it all the way in. These "holes" in our experiences become increasingly common as our mental state falls further into a state of disrepair.

If this hasn't happened to you personally, perhaps you've seen it happen to someone else. Whether it was a friend, a family member, a colleague, or a romantic partner, there is something particularly horrifying about seeing the light slowly slip away from someone's eyes when nothing is visibly, physically wrong with them. It looks like their soul is dying from the inside out.

This is what it looks like when the road of the mind begins to close.

It is not the presence of external stimuli but the mind's reaction to external stimuli that creates emotion and meaning. Nothing inherently feels like anything. Every spoken word, every touch, and every sensory experience that originates from outside of you must navigate the pathway of your mind before it means something to you. The deeper the ruts and potholes in the road of your mind, the more likely it is that external experiences get stuck on the way in. If you don't maintain this road carefully and repair it when it becomes damaged, you'll quickly find yourself numb and alone.

Picture a mile-long stretch of dead-end gravel road with deep ruts and grooves. At the end of this road is your inner, vulnerable self. Strewn along the road are vehicles that couldn't make it to you. The tow truck rusting in the ditch half a mile down the road is the love of a friend that couldn't quite get to you. The ambulance stuck in the giant puddle of mud is the concern of a family member who couldn't express themselves in a way that broke through your limiting belief systems about yourself. If you're anything like me, there's a veritable graveyard of missed connections between the outer world and your inner self.

The road is also responsible for taking what's inside of you and allowing it to be released out into the world, which is something nearly all of us want to do on at least some occasions. We long to be understood, and to do so we must share at least a portion of our story. We want our opinions, experiences, and beliefs to be valued and validated by others. Some of us want to create things that others can use or appreciate (like this book!). All these things must also travel the path of our minds. When that road falls into disrepair, everything stays stuck inside and nothing can get out.

I know this because it happened to me. My mental health declined so badly that the rest of the world fell away from me. I could still see everything life had to offer, just as I knew the hospital and the grocery story still existed even when our road was blocked growing up, but I had no way to access any of it. It was as if there was a six-inch-thick barrier of glass around me on all sides. I became trapped within myself. The only road connecting me to the rest of the world was blocked. I felt alone and isolated every day, no matter who I was with and what I was doing.

I longed to rejoin the world, but I didn't know how. Everything seemed so far away. Seeing the smiles and hearing the laughter of apparently normal people drove the point home further and further every day: You are not one of them. You're something else. Something that was never meant to be here. Something incomplete, unfinished.

The person I used to be is utterly unrecognizable to me today. I hardly spoke. When I walked, I looked straight down. When sitting or standing, I was rigid like a statue. I either slept constantly or went days on end without closing my eyes. My face had no expression. My voice had no intonation. On most days, I felt nothing but hopelessness, despair, and a longing to be anyone but myself. Simply continuing to live was a chore, an immense task that took everything I had in me on most days. My road was closed off.

Most people respond to this ever-growing sense of isolation and hopelessness by seeking a material solution outside of themselves. I know it's easy to believe that if you meet the right person, or have a child, or make more money these struggles would vanish. Don't get me wrong, these can be worthwhile pursuits, but they all have the same weakness regarding their ability to make your life better: Every one of them can be discredited and negated by an unhealthy and dysfunctional mind. When things are dark enough inside, none of these can get far enough in to produce any pleasant emotions.

Your mind filters and interprets everything around you. Let's say you're in a long-term, committed, healthy relationship with a partner who genuinely loves and appreciates you. That's wonderful, but if you're living with a deeply rooted belief that you're unlovable, you won't be able to feel any of it. Your beliefs about yourself will form a barrier that will block out every audible "I love you" and will tell you that every hug, every kiss, and every moment of intimacy are obligatory rather than genuine. The health of your mind will have an exponentially greater impact on how it feels to be alive every day than your partner will.

Your mind also serves as the author of the story of your life. It infers meaning from every experience you have. It translates impartial, disconnected experiences into a single, coherent narrative. It weaves certain types of experiences together to create the perception of a pattern while explaining away experiences that don't fit what it has decided is the trend.

Tell me if this pattern sounds familiar. When asked about your greatest mistakes or regrets, you can quickly and easily recall every failed test, every negative performance review, every instance of romantic rejection, and every other "lowlight" of your life. These moments feel like an interconnected set of experiences, chapters in a story that weave a consistent narrative. The narrative is one of inadequacy and shortcoming, and the main character is someone barely making it through life.

Conversely, when asked about your greatest successes or victories, you draw a blank or come up with only a few generic examples. You logically know that some parts of your life have been, and still are, good, but they feel like a series of disconnected events with no common thread tying them together. Your sense is that the best moments of your life are things that simply happened to you rather than things you caused to happen. Because you had nothing to do with them, they don't say anything about your ability or character; they were simply moments of good fortune. Only your negative experiences are integrated into the narrative of your life.

This common pattern shows the overwhelming damage caused by a mind that is constantly skewed towards the negative. As humans, we all tend to focus on the negatives to some degree, but for some of us, that point of view is constant and inescapable. Confirmation bias takes over, and we become unable to see ourselves clearly, locked inside our preexisting perceptions of our own identities. Even an overwhelming body of evidence to the contrary will not be enough to convince you that you aren't who you think you are because you'll simply explain it away. The only way to fix this mental glitch is to work on improving the health and functioning of your mind. It is our inner lives, not our outer lives, that create the deep, pervasive sense of happiness we long for.

Your mind is the most enduring worldly possession you will ever own, the only true constant from birth to death. Think about how much time you spend in an average year taking care of your house. If you add up all of the chores (the cleaning, the organizing, and the decluttering), it's almost certainly hundreds of hours even if you aren't ultra picky about your home environment. How does this compare to the amount of time you spend in an average year taking care of your mind? The vast majority of us spend more time on our homes, but this is ultimately an inefficient use of resources. Doesn't it make more sense to allocate your time and energy based on how long something will be a part of your life? You probably won't live in your current home for the rest of your life, but you will undeniably inhabit your mind until the day you die. Unless cyborgs.

Our minds do not naturally maintain themselves. Just like our bodies, they accumulate damage and injuries as we navigate a challenging and broken world. Minor injuries heal naturally without intervention, but severe injuries can permanently change our functioning. Just as with a broken leg or a torn tendon, experiences like trauma, betrayal, and grief can permanently change how we navigate this life, if they aren't treated with care and support.

When you were younger, it was the responsibility of those around you to provide you with this care. Whether they managed their obligations to you with respect and compassion or grudging obligation, none of us make it into adulthood unscathed. The only person who can maintain the road that is your mind is you. You are the engineer, the construction crew, and the snow removal team, all at once. If you don't maintain this road, it will become so uneven, so neglected, and so impassable that you'll end up trapped within yourself. It won't matter what's happening outside of you because you won't be able to access it. The best this life has to offer will feel like nothing at all. You won't have the motivation, the courage, or the coherence to share your inner experience with others. When that happens, you will feel like I once did: as if you're surrounded by a glass enclosure that makes the rest of the world feel abstract, intangible, and ultimately inaccessible.

Even spiritual relationships can be damaged or blocked by an unhealthy mind. The notion of any kind of creator or designer making your life or the world you inhabit becomes a lot less appealing when you despise all of it. When I was at my lowest, I could not feel anyone or anything loving me, or even fathom the idea of it. I hated myself and my life so much that it seemed only logical that everyone else hated me, too. I wasn't open to any kind of meaningful relationship with anyone, human or otherwise, until I began to address my inner pain. It was so immense that it blocked out everything else.

During my darkest times, I would have told you that anyone who created me must have been a sadist. It was part of why I resented my parents for a time; as they were my worldly creators, I viewed them as partially responsible for my pain and expected them to somehow fix it, which of course they could not. And if some kind of God or deity had a hand in my creation, I would have told you that I hated them, too.

These feelings did not accurately reflect reality. My family did still love me, and I'm pretty sure some of my friends did, too. But I couldn't feel it, couldn't believe in it. If you believe in any kind of a God, there's no logical reason to believe that God's love is withdrawn when you are physically or mentally unwell. It just feels that way because you become less aware of it and less able to access it. Your awareness of it can be blocked, cutting you off from spiritual love.

For all of these reasons, the first and most fundamental lesson I want to teach you from my own life is this: Begin within. Take excellent care of your mind, because it's the only thing connecting you to everything else you care about in this world.

The Application

How to Care for Yourself

There are four basic resources your mind needs to remain healthy and functional: blood, oxygen, caloric energy, and rest. Blood and oxygen are provided by the heart and the lungs. Caloric energy comes from consistently having food in your digestive system. Rest comes from sleep and breaks from stress. This is but a taste of the sage-like wisdom I'll be imparting upon you during our time together.

In all seriousness, if you're able to consistently provide your brain with the resources it needs to be healthy, that alone will solve a lot of your problems. This might sound like a tremendously oversimplified solution to a seemingly insurmountable problem that has plagued you for your entire adult life, and possibly even before then, but so few people consistently meet these needs for themselves. Have you ever experienced a sustained period in your life when your physical activity level, sleeping habits, and nutritional patterns (including intake of substances like caffeine and alcohol) were all in a good place at the same time? I'm betting that your answer is either "No" or "Yes, and it was the period of my life when I felt like I was at my best." That's not a coincidence.

Your mind functions on a system quite like the power grids that underlie most large cities. In the event of a power shortage or outage, certain high-priority systems are kept online at all costs to prevent catastrophic failure. Facilities such as hospitals and water treatment plants receive top priority, since the residents of the city cannot survive or function for long without the services these facilities provide. Other less critical structures, such as stores and restaurants, might stay dark until the power system is fully back online.

Blood, oxygen, caloric energy, and rest collectively form the power supply of your mind. If any of these resources are in short supply, some of your mental functions become less active. Within the power grid of your mind, the highest-priority systems are your basic physiological functions. Your heart needs to keep beating and your lungs need to keep breathing. Your ability to intake basic sensory inputs (sight, sound, taste, touch, and smell) is also critical for survival. All of these capabilities reside in your hindbrain. Your hindbrain will receive ample resources no matter how exhausted or malnourished you become, because if it doesn't you will literally die in a matter of minutes. It would be pretty stupid of your brain to let that happen, and despite how frustrating your brain can be sometimes, it is anything but stupid.

Your primitive survival responses are nearly as integral to your continued existence. The ability to generate emotions such as fear, anger, and pleasure is essential to mobilizing survival-oriented behaviors. Your ability to enter a fight-or-flight response allows you to react instinctively to potential threats. All of these capabilities reside in your midbrain. Your midbrain will almost never get cut off from necessary resources either, because while you will not immediately perish without these skills, you won't be long for this world. Being unable to sense danger or feel sadness or anger would get you into trouble very quickly.

The part of your mind that takes the biggest hit when any resource falls below optimal levels is your prefrontal cortex. You can technically live without a functioning prefrontal cortex indefinitely if someone else is managing your basic needs. Babies barely have one at all when they're first born. The prefrontal cortex is responsible for, among other things:

- Keeping you calm and composed during challenging situations;
- Helping you tell the difference between good ideas and bad ideas;
- Correctly interpreting and responding to subtle social cues like tone of voice and body language;
- Stopping you from doing things that feel good in the moment but really screw up your life later;
- Making and following through with long-term plans;
- Helping you keep your attention on things that are important but not necessarily interesting or stimulating.

Are these the areas of life where you struggle the most? If so, we've localized your problem. Your prefrontal cortex isn't functioning properly, and we need to direct more resources towards it. If we can get your brain working right, *all* of those things get dramatically better. Trying to navigate this harsh, confusing, impersonal world without a properly resourced prefrontal cortex can feel a bit like trying to mow your lawn with scissors. Even if you're pushing yourself as hard as you possibly can day after day, you just aren't going to get very far without the right tool. Keeping your brain stocked with everything it needs to function optimally is like trading in those scissors for a riding mower. The difference will be immense. The difficulty level of enjoying life will decline from "impossible" to "quite difficult." Progress!

If you have never simultaneously been able to achieve good sleeping habits, nutritional habits, and physical activity habits, you have no idea what your mind is capable of. It's always been facing at least one resource constraint that has massively impaired its performance. Any beliefs you have formed about your competency or your capability during periods of resource constraint should be discarded due to being formed by data collected under faulty circumstances. You are almost certainly dramatically smarter, more capable, and more resilient than you've previously experienced yourself to be.

A brain without a fully operational prefrontal cortex functions quite similarly to a workplace without an effective manager. Panic ensues anytime a new task or responsibility is introduced because nobody knows who is in charge of what. Who is going to do this? And when? And how? Lots of time is wasted doing absolutely nothing. There's no real sense of guidance or direction. It's a chaotic, unpleasant place to spend time.

This is one of my biggest criticisms of modern psychotherapy. There is a strong emphasis on learning and practicing coping skills for distress, which in and of itself is valuable, but minimal emphasis on assessing whether an individual's mind is physically healthy enough to cope with distress. If your prefrontal cortex is barely working, it's mostly irrelevant how knowledgeable you are about what you should do during stressful situations, because you won't be able to access and apply that knowledge. Management style is irrelevant if the manager has been on vacation for a decade.

Conversely, when your prefrontal cortex is working properly, many of your distressing emotions will be regulated automatically.

Concerns and problems that have little to no basis in reality will be filtered out as illogical or irrelevant. Only the pressing, objectively important issues will make it to your consciousness. The rest will simply die out below the surface. Believe it or not, your mind isn't supposed to automatically torture you endlessly over every social miscue or unfinished task, nor is it supposed to panic over every unexpected challenge or minor change of plans.

Being in possession of a healthy brain will not automatically solve all of your problems, but it will make it possible for you to solve them. Let's review in more detail what exactly is required to finally give your mind everything it needs to do its job properly.

Rest

There are two types of rest: physical and mental. Understanding how to get both is critical, and providing one while neglecting the other will leave you stuck. For my readers who also happen to be gamers, the two types of rest function very similarly to the systems found in role-playing games where characters have both health and mana reserves. You need to manage both resources effectively to survive, and if either is depleted, you'll quickly find yourself in trouble.

Physical rest comes primarily from getting an adequate amount of high-quality sleep. The average adult needs eight hours of sleep per night, and 98 percent of all adults need somewhere between seven and a half and eight and a half hours of sleep, so you most likely fall within that range. If you're used to getting significantly more or less than that, your mind and body can adapt to these conditions and you might feel "OK" most of the time, but you will never be at 100 percent if you're oversleeping or under sleeping. Please be aware that you might briefly experience a confusing increase in fatigue and decrease in cognitive performance when you finally start getting the right amount of sleep. Your brain can get so used to functioning on a maladaptive quantity of rest that it can take a few days for it to respond correctly to finally having its needs met. This is a temporary adjustment to your sleep efficiency, and it should only last a few days, so just power through it.

However, getting adequate sleep is a matter of both quantity and quality. Not all sleep is created equal. You move through the various cycles that comprise a full night of sleep more efficiently if you sleep at the same time every night. And "night" simply refers to when you sleep, not necessarily when it happens to be dark out. It really doesn't matter when you sleep if you're able to be consistent with it and it works for your lifestyle. Pick a sleep time and a wake time, and do your best to stick to them as close to seven days a week as possible. If you allow yourself to sleep on the days when you don't have something you need to wake up early for (likely weekends), your sleep schedule starts to shift, and you end up feeling a bit jetlagged when you have to wake up early once again.

Practicing effective sleep hygiene can also improve the quality of your sleep. Try to avoid caffeine within ten hours of bedtime and alcohol within six hours of bedtime, as both substances negatively impact your ability to reach deeper stages of sleep, which is necessary for a sense of being well rested the following day. Make sure your sleeping environment is quiet, dark, and cool, and try to stay out of it when you aren't actively trying to sleep.

We rest mentally by getting a break from the crushing worldly stress most of us are under at all times. Sleeping is not a mentally restful activity because you aren't conscious to experience it. If you're skeptical of this, consider the following scenario: You work sixteen hours a day, but you get eight hours of consistent, high-quality sleep every night. If the job is not physically demanding, your body could probably manage this schedule, but your mind would be in rough shape.

In order to experience a true break from the stressors of life, we need to spend time every day on activities that are high stimulation, low stress, and at least somewhat novel. These three variables comprise the active ingredients of effective mental rest.

High-stimulation activities are those that command your attention to a near-complete degree. When you're engaged in something stimulating, you think about very little else because your mind is fully engaged with the present task. Your problems temporarily seem to melt away because what you're doing takes everything your brain has to offer, and there simply isn't any attention left over to worry with. The stimulation value of an activity varies tremendously from person to person, so I can't tell you exactly what activities will meet these criteria for you. What you want to avoid are the low-engagement, "mindless" activities we tend to gravitate towards when we're stressed. These seem appealing because we "turn our brains off," but that's exactly what we need to stay away from when we need a break. Because these activities require little from you, they don't effectively get your mind off the stressors of your day, and you'll notice that your thoughts keep drifting back to problems and concerns, robbing you of the break you desperately need.

Low-stress activities are behaviors you engage in just for the sake of doing them. It doesn't matter to you how well you perform or whether you produce something of value, you just want to do the activity. As soon as you start to heap performance expectations upon an activity, it just becomes another stressor. If you can't draw without critiquing your art, drawing is not low stress for you. If you can't watch sports without being upset if your team loses, sports are not low stress for you. If even your hobbies are stressful and you're unable to detach your emotions from the outcome, you'll never get a break. Your life simply becomes an endless loop of trading work stress for other stress and is critically devoid of periods where you are conscious and awake but not experiencing stress. This will slowly grind you down even if you happen to be sleeping fine.

You'll need to switch up these activities from time to time in order to keep them novel. When an activity loses its novelty value, your mind begins to automate the steps involved, and it ceases to be mentally engaging. Think of the difference between the first time you drove somewhere and the hundredth time you drove to the same place. Once you've more or less mastered the route, you stop paying conscious attention to driving, and your mind is free to wander to other things. That wandering works against us here because it's likely to wander back to stressors.

Caloric Energy

Your brain lacks a stomach. It does not have the capacity to store caloric energy, and it's only able to access whatever is in your bloodstream at any given time. Eating a reasonably well-proportioned and balanced meal gives your mind fuel for about six waking hours, so you should try to avoid going longer than that without eating. This might mean you sometimes need to pack snacks for yourself before leaving the house, like you're a toddler about to embark on a field trip. Taking excellent care of your mind is not always glamorous work.

A well-proportioned meal is one that is neither too small nor too large. There isn't an exact number of calories or ounces you need to consume, and getting rigid or perfectionistic about this will work against you here. The last thing you want is for food to become yet another stressor. Instead of turning meals into a calculus problem, try to eat at a relatively slow pace and work on intuitively gauging your fullness by paying attention to your internal physical sensations. Try to stop eating just before you feel full because there's a bit of lag time between our sense of satiety and the amount of food we've consumed.

If the meal is too small, your mind won't get a full six hours of energy from it, and you'll be riding an emotional and cognitive roller coaster until your next meal as your blood sugar spikes and drops. If the meal is too large, your body mobilizes additional blood flow to your metabolic system to assist with breaking it down. Want to guess where some of that blood comes from? The prefrontal cortex. That's the real reason you feel tired after a large meal (no, Uncle Barry, it isn't the tryptophan in the turkey; you just ate too much food).

You should also try to consume a reasonable balance of protein, carbohydrates, and dietary fats at every meal. Protein mostly comes from meat, fish, some dairy, and some plant-based sources such as tofu. Dietary fats can be found in butter, oil, nuts and nut butters, cream, and avocados. Carbohydrates come mostly from bread, pasta, rice, and fruits and vegetables. This is obviously not an exhaustive list, just a brief overview of the categories of food that should be on your plate every meal.

Try to avoid fad diets and other nutritional "hacks." In addition to generally not being optimal for your mental functioning, most of them are unsustainable for long periods of time, so even if they did produce some benefit, it would only be temporary. I'm also not a big fan of fasting, as the research on it with regard to individuals who have mood or anxiety disorders is too inconsistent for my liking. Fasting also seems to be motivated typically by weight-loss aspirations, which are often detrimental to your mental health.

Blood and Oxygen

Though technically separate resources, blood and oxygen are combined here because they are optimized through the same action: regular physical activity. This tends to be the tallest hurdle you'll need to clear on the quest for a healthy mind. Many popular workout routines and programs call for a level of physical activity that is well beyond what our minds need us to do in order to stay mentally healthy. This, unfortunately, results in a lot of people pushing themselves too hard, burning out, and giving up.

According to meta-analyses (studies of studies) on physical activity and mental performance, three to five days a week of exercise is plenty. The ideal duration of these workouts is between twenty and forty minutes long. If you don't mind doing longer workouts, you can get away with doing them less often. If you prefer shorter workouts, try to do them more frequently. Maxing out both of these, e.g., five days a week for forty minutes, is almost certainly unnecessary if the purpose of your physical activity is to support your mental health.

The mental health benefits of physical activity appear to max out at moderate intensity. The intensity of a workout is partially determined by your current fitness level, so if you're just getting started it won't take much to get you there. You can gauge the intensity of a workout by how you feel. If you notice a little bit of skin sweat, a discernable increase in heart rate, and a slight shortness of breath, you're right where you want to be. If you're drenched in sweat, your heart is pounding, and you'd need to catch your breath to talk you've overdone it, so cool it, Goggins.

The format of exercise seems to be irrelevant as long as your workout meets the aforementioned criteria. As a certified hater of all things cardio, this was one of the most liberating pieces of synthesized research I have ever read. Whatever type of exercise you happen to enjoy, just do that! If you don't enjoy any of it, do whatever you hate the least. If you really can't think of anything you wouldn't mind doing regularly, you need to expand your horizons a bit as there are some truly niche workouts out there. You might be the next hobby-horsing champion in waiting.

It's worth noting that pushing yourself too far beyond these parameters isn't just a matter of diminishing returns; it may actually be detrimental to your mental health. The relationship between physical exercise and brain functioning is an inverted bell curve, meaning that spending hours in the gym ripping yourself a new one every day basically comes full circle and is just as bad for you as not exercising at all, so if you're that A++++, extra credit, 110 percent type of person, you're going to need to really rein in those tendencies here. Also, calm down.

My anecdotal experience also supports this finding. I fell into a deep obsession with the gym and my body for about a year, and it was one of the most dysfunctional and unhappy years of my life. I hyper-analyzed myself in the mirror every day, counted calories religiously, and completely systematized my workouts. I'm very thankful I didn't have access to anabolic steroids because I definitely would have taken them. Sorry for that unexpectedly dark detour from what had previously been a relatively light and humorous three paragraphs.

If the parameters I've outlined here feel daunting to you, I have two recommendations. The first is to approach your goals in a stepwise manner rather than expecting yourself to immediately get to the top of your game. The patterns of sleeping, eating, and moving described in this chapter represent the optimal habits in each of these domains. If you're currently a long way off from those benchmarks, set some intermediate goals that you think you can meet in a month or two so that you can enjoy a tangible sense of progression and reward, rather than expecting yourself to magically become a completely different person tomorrow than the one you've been every day until now.

The second is to save increasing physical activity for last. It's not any less important than rest or nutrition; it's just a lot harder to achieve when you aren't getting enough of those things. Regular physical activity is a difficult thing to do for most people even under the best of circumstances, and it becomes exponentially more difficult when you're feeling tired, hungry, or both. Making improvements in sleep and nutrition first should give you an extra boost of energy and motivation, which you can then invest in regular physical activity.

Once you're able to do all of these things with reasonable consistency, you will be in possession of a physically healthy brain, possibly for the first time in your life. This already puts you among rare company, and it *will* make a noticeable difference in how you feel. This is how I live every day of my life, and I believe with all of my heart that these habits are the single biggest reason I am no longer the person I described in the introduction of this book. For some people, this may be all that is needed to turn your life around. However, if your brain is anything like mine, these habits are necessary but not sufficient. It's going to take more. A lot more.

Truth Two

Envy Is Ignorance

The Story

The Lake

The splash was so loud I thought someone had died. My sister was crying. My brother was hyperventilating. My mom was panicking. I couldn't piece together what had just happened.

We had all been fishing together in our favorite bay. Even though it was straight across the water from our house it felt like entering another world. There were no houses or roads on that side of the lake, so the whole area felt much wilder and more primitive than on our relatively developed shore. There was an underwater island centered within the bay where the water was only a few feet deep, and we could easily see all the way down to the bottom. Surrounding the island was a rapidly sloping drop-off where the vibrant, lush green of the lake bottom descended eerily into an impenetrable darkness within a foot or two. For as long as I can recall, looking into the dark part of the water gave me an ominous feeling. I always wondered if something was looking back at me from just beyond where I could see.

That foot or two of "in-between" space was where the best fishing was. We could almost, but not quite, see the bottom. Tendrils of weeds and cabbage sprung up from lake floor, creating fractals and patterns that twisted into unseen depths. The holes between the weeds always held fish. We loved to drop our neon lures into these holes and wait for them to disappear, the telltale sign that they were now inside the mouth of an unseen fish waiting just beyond where we could see. The mystery and excitement of reeling in with no idea what was on the other end was exhilarating and addictive to me. It made the anxiety of sitting next to the foreboding darkness of the drop-off tolerable.

Strange things tended to happen to us in the bay. It was our lake's version of the Bermuda Triangle. There was a school of what had to be over a thousand ciscoes, silvery baitfish that seemed to swim endlessly in circles, constantly suspending just above the drop-off. Right around sunset, the entire school would sometimes leap violently from the water in unison, giving the surface of the lake the appearance of a pot of boiling water. Our mother theorized that something was chasing the ciscoes and causing them to panic, but we never saw anything following them. I found it incredibly disturbing to think that anything could scare fish so badly that they would flee to a place they couldn't breathe just to get away.

The other mystery of the bay was the splashing. Fish jump from time to time, turtles and frogs hop into the lake from shore, and waterbirds land, so splashing is a common enough sound on a lake, but this wasn't the sound of any of those things. It was something louder, more aggressive, and seemingly much larger. We thought it might be a beaver slapping its tail on the water, warning us to stay out of its territory, but we had never seen a beaver in the bay and beavers aren't exactly renowned for their stealth and subtlety. There also weren't any lodges or dams on that part of the lake, so I was always skeptical of the beaver hypothesis.

Many lessons in the wilderness are learned the hard way, and figuring out the best way for three excitable, impulsive children to simultaneously fish out of a fourteen-foot boat was one of them. When all of us were trying to cast lures, hooks would whizz by faces like bullets, sometimes coming within inches of eyes, ears, and noses. We miraculously managed to avoid hooking each other, but our mother's expensive prescription glasses did nobly sacrifice themselves to save her left eye on one occasion. Thankfully, the casting drama mostly ended when we discovered dangling.

Because the lake was so clear, if we were fishing somewhere shallow, we could just look down into the lake and find fish. Once we spotted one, we'd drop the lure straight down into the water, skipping the process of casting entirely. We called this style of fishing "dangling," partially because that's what we would do with our lures, but also because it's what we would do with our legs. Dangling was most fun when we sat in a row on the side of the boat with our spindly little appendages hanging inches above the water. We felt more connected to the lake when we did this, and it added an extra layer of visceral excitement. Having all the human weight on one side of the boat caused it to angle sharply towards the water, giving us the constant feeling that we were on the verge of falling in. Sometimes our toes would even dip into the cold water on windy days.

Dangling worked best on "glass" days. That's what we called it when the sun was shining and the wind was a whisper. With no waves to disrupt the surface of the water, glass is exactly what the lake looked like. It perfectly reflected the ring of evergreen trees surrounding the lake and the deep-blue sky above and, more importantly, we could see even farther down into the water than when the chop of the waves divided the surface. The closest comparison I can provide to looking down into the water on a glass day is looking at the night sky on a cloudless summer evening out in the country. It's absolutely stunning. Glass days were our favorite days to dangle, and this was a perfect glass day. I knew it from the second I opened my eyes and looked out our bedroom window to see the big white pine motionless and unbothered by the wind. Dangling in the bay was all I could think about that morning.

My siblings had been fishing on one side of the boat while I was trying the opposite side. Our mother was up front, keeping us right on the drop-off where the fish were. Then I heard the splash. The familiar sound that echoed across the bay from time to time, but this time much louder, much closer. It sounded as if it was inches away. My first thought was that one of my siblings had accidentally knocked the other into the lake, but when I spun around to see what happened, they were both still sitting on the edge of the boat like nothing happened. Then I realized how still they were. Unusually still, as if they were frozen. And they weren't fishing.

That's when my sister started to cry. It wasn't a normal cry. It was a scream cry, a cry of fear rather than sadness. A sound I had never heard come out of her before. Our mom kept asking her what had happened, wanting desperately to provide comfort or reassurance but not knowing how. She was just as in the dark as I was about what, exactly, had just happened.

Finally, my brother spoke. His voice was ragged with adrenaline and every word seemed to require unimaginable effort to force out of his hyperventilating body. "It was . . . it was a . . . a musky! And . . . it was *huge*! And it . . . it tried to . . . to eat Alison's fish!"

Now I understood. Not just what happened seconds ago to cause the chaos, but every mystery of the bay that had left us baffled for years. Moments before the splash, my sister had been lifting a small sunfish out of the water to unhook it. She was blissfully unaware that the fish she had hooked was being watched. A massive predator fish had been stalking it from the depths, waiting for the right moment to strike. When my sister pulled the fish from the water with her rod, the sudden movement triggered the predator fish's prey drive. It rushed to the surface at full speed and launched itself fully out of the water, inches from her face, in a desperate attempt to catch its unexpectedly fleet lunch.

Muskellunge were practically an urban legend on our lake. We had read stories about their size and ferocity, but we had never actually seen one before that day. We heard that they grew to sizes exponentially bigger than anything we had caught. They were also said to be relatively unafraid of humans and would sometimes approach swimmers and boats with curiosity instead of darting away out of fear as most fish do when they encounter people. Everything I knew about them made them seem like something that didn't belong in a lake. Anything that big and aggressive should be relegated to the oceans with the sharks.

We quickly motored back home to gather our nerves, quite finished with fishing for the rest of the day. According to my siblings, this fish lived up to every seemingly implausible description of a musky we had been told about. My sister, nine years old at the time, said the fish was bigger than her. Its mouth was said to have held a row of serrated teeth that resembled a bread knife. My brother mentioned something about a "dark" look in its eyes that he couldn't quite articulate. Apparently, this thing was pure nightmare fuel.

Muskies are relatively territorial, especially the larger, older fish. If they find a consistent source of food in an area where they feel comfortable and secure, they typically make that area their home and don't stray far from it. This musky had almost certainly been the unseen predator haunting the ciscoes in the evening and the source of the mysterious splashing that would echo across the bay from time to time. Even though we had never seen it before that day, it had probably been lurking within casting distance of our boat for years, hidden just beyond where we could see.

My sister named this fish "Nemesis." We told stories about him, made drawings of him. He became an almost mythological figure in our family, a cryptid come to life in front of our eyes on a random glass afternoon. Although we never saw him again after that day, our awareness of his presence changed things.

We didn't really dangle anymore. We would still occasionally fish without casting, but sitting on the edge of the boat with our toes inches from the water no longer felt like innocent, harmless fun. I tried it once and couldn't stop envisioning Nemesis rushing up from the depths to bite my foot off because he mistook my toes for ciscoes.

We still loved fishing, but it felt different. There was always a hint of nervousness, even when fishing outside the bay, as we wondered if we might catch a glimpse of another sea monster. We reeled our fish in a little bit faster, yanking them from unseen jaws below the surface. Once I hooked something clearly much larger than our usual sunfish and perch, and when my father came over to help me I shoved the rod into his hands and ran to the back of the boat, terrified to look at what was on the end of my lure and thoroughly convinced I had accidentally hooked into Nemesis (it was a three-pound bass).

For me, it also created a lot of existential concerns. I wondered if anything in life was as happy, idyllic, and carefree as it seemed, or if everything was like the bay, haunted by an unseen predator lurking just beyond my perception. Was there always darkness below the surface? Was everything being chased by something?

For the first time in our lives, we finally had confirmation of something we had always sensed: Monsters really did lurk in the darkness.

The Lesson

Nemesis

Perpetually lurking beneath the surface in my mind is the possibility that my life is dramatically and irreversibly worse than someone else's. I used to dream about waking up in another life, another place, another time, or another body. Other people seemed so vibrant, so interesting, so full of purpose and value. They had friends, achievements, and ambitions. I had video games, Hamburger Helper, and staring out my window.

My envy for the lives of other people was often what stopped me from trying to improve my own life. I felt sure that no matter what I did, I could never have what they had and could never feel what they felt. Investing time and energy into myself was a fruitless endeavor, like throwing my pennies into a black hole rather than a wishing well.

I made up ridiculous stories about my background to try and seem like a more interesting person, although I'm sure it was obvious to anyone who had the misfortune of listening to me that I was just making things up. During one particularly low season of life, I would download pictures of obscure metal musicians and use them to catfish AOL chat rooms, desperate for just a hint of validation that I was an interesting, meaningful, attractive person. It's a truly disheartening feeling to have 100 percent of your self-esteem come from stolen valor.

Unsurprisingly, none of this behavior made me feel any better about myself for more than five minutes. In fact, the more focused I became on what other people had that I lacked, the more I hated myself and my own existence. I was stuck in a feedback loop that didn't appear to have an escape. It felt like everyone other than me had been handed some kind of instruction manual on how to operate a human life while I couldn't even figure out how to get the stupid thing to turn on.

I realize now that every single person I fantasized about being had their own Nemesis. Most of the relationships that looked so healthy and desirable to me have crashed and burned in dramatic fashion. Many of my heroes have died from suicide or overdoses. I've come to understand that so much of the excitement and achievement I once envied with every neurotransmitter of my broken brain was just a struggling person trying desperately to fill the void of an absent parent or escape the memory of some horrific trauma. The people whose lives I wanted so badly to escape into were just as tormented as me. They were simply far better at masking it.

For the most part, we can only see into the shallows of how others think, feel, and live. Most people put the best parts of their lives on display in the most visible locations, like social media and other public spaces, and keep their personal darkness hidden out of sight. Our minds have a hard time understanding that what's hidden in the depths can look dramatically different than what's right below the surface. We look at the first ten feet of something that's one hundred feet deep and assume that the unseen matches the seen. Our own existence, so full of flaws and seeming to constantly fluctuate between overwhelmingly stressful and unbearably understimulating, seems miserable by contrast.

What looks desirable and beautiful often has something terrible lurking beneath. You may see signs of a monster bubbling up every now and then, the baitfish being chased by the nightmare below, but rarely, if ever, will you fully witness someone else's Nemesis. This universal human instinct to mask shame, failure, and trauma can lead you to believe you're alone in your struggles. Nothing could be further from the truth. Everyone is being silently stalked by something.

Put slightly less eloquently, you know everything that sucks about being you. You only have this level of information about yourself. You don't know what sucks about being someone else. But I promise you, something does. Probably many things.

As a therapist, I spend much of my day talking with people about what they feel is missing from their lives. It's so tempting to think that the object of our current focus is the final step on our journey to feeling happy and complete. When you've conducted as many therapy sessions as I have, you eventually realize how cyclical most of our desires are. The following is a dramatized aggregation of many clients I've worked with over the years, but my days often look a bit like this:

My first client of the day has a good support network and ample free time to pursue her many passions. She's a talented artist with incredible insights, but she lost her job six months ago and is hurtling towards poverty at an alarming rate. She struggles to use her downtime for leisure or productivity, instead spending large chunks of her day waist-deep in regret. She wishes she could go back in time and slap herself into opening a savings account instead of making so many impulse purchases and ordering delivery for every dinner for months.

She feels needy, desperate, and pathetic. She just wishes she had a decent job and enough money to pay her bills.

My second client of the day is doing well financially. He skipped a grade in high school and breezed through college because of natural intellect. With a high skill level in a growing industry, he easily obtained a high-paying position in his field, but he has next to no meaningful human interaction outside of his workplace. The few friends he made in high school scattered to various out-of-state universities and haven't come back. He is at least a decade younger than any of his colleagues at the small business he works for. Although he exchanges the usual greetings with them every day, the interactions are painfully superficial. His ongoing isolation has him thoroughly convinced that he is unlikable, rejected, and broken. He just wishes he could find a friend with shared hobbies and passions.

My third client of the day has a great group of friends. She gets together multiple nights per week with them to watch their favorite "trashy" reality TV shows and gossip, and they have two or three annual weekend getaways for concerts and spa days. Although she loves her friends dearly, she grows lonelier and sadder by the day because she longs for a romantic partner. She's been single for years and is starting to worry that "years" could easily become "forever." Her days are fraught with despair that it's too late, her time has passed, and nobody will find her interesting or attractive in that way for the rest of her life. She feels ugly, old, and hopeless. She just wishes she could feel a deep, intimate connection to one person.

My fourth client of the day just celebrated his tenth anniversary with his wife. They're an incredibly photogenic couple who could probably model for Ralph Lauren. He has a good job, and he's been climbing the corporate ladder consistently for years. However, coming home to his wife and their dog feels more and more depressing after every miscarriage. They've been trying to conceive for years and have never made it out of the first trimester. Every one of those losses was a devastating heartbreak, and neither he nor his wife are sure if they can handle another one. They're terrified to keep trying but equally terrified to stop trying. Most of his friends have children now, and their social outings tend to be confined to children's spaces and activities, so he's usually not invited. He knows he's with the right person, but he can't imagine a happy future without biological children of his own. He feels lost, purposeless, and disconnected. He just wants to come home to a crying baby to hold.

My fifth client of the day has a surplus of children. Five, to be exact, ranging in age from four to sixteen. All five are physically and mentally healthy. They are passionate, active children with a wide range of interests including athletics, music, and drama. Every waking hour of my client's life is fully consumed by parenting duties. She cherishes every precious second she has to herself and longs for space to breathe. Although she loves her children, she feels trapped, burdened, and stuck. She just wants to run away and have no obligations or responsibilities, even if it means living with nothing.

Let me be clear on this: I am not belittling any of these concerns. Finances, friends, romantic love, children, and free time can all have a tremendous impact on the quality of our lives, but if they were truly "the secret" to fulfillment, nobody who had those things would be unhappy with life. I've worked with people in every possible life circumstance, from those without a place to call home to wildly successful entrepreneurs who have more money and fame than I can comprehend, and one thing they all have in common is a longing for something that someone else has.

I know you feel like it would be different for you. You're well aware that not everyone who has what you so desperately long for is happy, but that's because they don't appreciate it like you would. They haven't struggled for it the way you have. The object of your desire simply fell into their lap without years or decades of pursuit, without sacrifice and sobbing, without pain and heartbreak, so of course it doesn't make them happy. If they knew half of the hardships you've been through, they'd wake up every day with a smile on their face. I know you believe this with all your heart, but that's just not how brains work.

As a doctoral student, I spent several years working at a beautiful, impeccably run private practice. The owner of the practice, a psychologist named Kim, embodied everything I wanted to be as a professional. She was brilliant yet easy to talk to, firm and direct yet kind. When she spoke people listened, not out of fear for their jobs but out of respect for her insights. Her practice doubled in size during the three years I worked for her. She had a seemingly endless wait list of therapy clients and divided her time evenly between direct clinical work and business operations. Nearly every time she ran a group with me, at least one of the clients would have a tear-filled breakthrough. I used to just stare at Kim sometimes and think about how incredible it must feel every day to wake up and be her.

After leaving that practice and starting my job as a hospital psychologist, I still felt like I was constantly in her shadow, even though we rarely spoke to one another and practiced in different states. Lurking under every achievement, every promotion, and every successful presentation was a thought I couldn't escape: *Kim is still better.* She was the benchmark I was aiming for, and I knew I could never be satisfied until I made it. I'd seen what it was possible for a therapist to be, and I couldn't accept anything less than that from myself.

Now, as the owner of a midsized private practice that is growing rapidly, the supervisor of several young up-and-coming clinicians, and a therapist with an absurdly long wait list, I realized something the other day: I have basically become Kim with a YouTube channel. That realization snuck up on me because I most certainly do not feel the way I imagined Kim must feel on a normal day of life. I still just feel like me, with my normal ups and downs, wins and losses, triumphs and doubts. I'll never be Kim, but I don't think Kim was ever Kim either. The picture in my mind, the person I was trying to become, didn't really exist.

This constant pattern of achievement followed by disappointment continues because we devalue things almost immediately after obtaining them. What we're missing always feels so much more important than what we have. Whether it's people, pets, status, degrees, achievements, or possessions, almost everyone's life is littered with former "missing pieces" that suddenly don't seem quite as special once they stop being missing. When we finally get what we've been chasing for so long and it still doesn't make us feel whole, we usually conclude that we were focused on the wrong piece, recalibrate, and try again. It's so hard for us to accept that the entire model of happiness and satisfaction we're all operating under is deeply flawed.

This endless drive to reach some arbitrary next level is nothing more than an outdated mammalian survival response. It wasn't that long ago that humans had to do things like store food for winter or times of famine. We are literally designed to feel like nothing we have is ever good enough so that we don't accidentally die of complacency. As social animals with a penchant for comparative analysis, we can be feeling pretty good about our stash of potatoes until we sneak a peek into our neighbor's storehouse and see that he has about 25 percent more potatoes than we do, causing us to emotionally spiral out of newfound fear that we don't have enough potatoes.

Basically, you're unhappy with your life because your great, great, great, great grandfather Henry didn't grow enough potatoes and accidentally introduced permanent existential dread into your family DNA. Thanks a freaking lot, Henry.

We're all just participants in one giant experiment where we move the pieces of our respective lives around a little, trade one thing for another, then assess the results to see if we feel any happier after doing so. That other person's life that you think makes yours look boring, unimportant, or unfulfilling does not exist in objective reality. You have no idea how other people feel, what they think, or how they live. You don't know what they've given up to get what they have, and in some cases you don't even know if what they claim to have is real. You're chasing a surface-level impression of something that runs so much deeper than you realize. You will never find peace and contentment in this world if you don't learn to love your own waters.

The Application

Celebrate, Identify, Locate, Pursue

You will never catch the feelings you've been chasing if you keep pursuing the lives other people appear to be living. This thought process keeps you trapped on an endless roller coaster of envy and meaninglessness. You need to stop looking at them and start looking at yourself.

I know. Stop cringing and just listen.

First, indulge me in a little experiment. Pull up whichever social media account you're most active on and look at your photos, your reels, your posts, and any other content you share with the world. Pretend for a moment that this isn't your account. Look at it as if it were the account of a stranger. Without knowing everything happening behind the scenes, what do you think of this person's life?

It looks pretty good, doesn't it?

I figured out this trick last year. I was sitting in my backyard on a warm summer evening after a very difficult day at work. A few weeks earlier, a cyberattack had completely disrupted our revenue stream. We hadn't seen a penny since then. Everything was "stuck" in "the system" somewhere. I'd burned through all my savings and had another payroll cycle coming up the following day. My only options for paying my employees were to dip into my 401(k), take out a loan, or use the money I had saved up for taxes and kick that can down the road.

In between perseverating on all my problems, stressors, and challenges, I happened to look up and see my daughter on the swing set going higher than she ever had before. I took a quick fifteen-second video to commemorate the achievement, posted it on social media, and then returned to my rumination.

The following day I was scrolling through my feed and came across a video that stopped me. It was a reel of a perfect day in a beautiful backyard. The sun was out, the wind was gently blowing the leaves, and songbirds were serenading. There was a little girl on a wooden swing set about the same age as my daughter. She had a giant grin plastered across her face, clearly pleased with herself as her hair whipped around with every swinging motion. I thought whoever took this video must have a wonderful life. Everything looked so sublime, picturesque, and carefree.

It took me a couple of seconds to realize I was watching my own video. My reaction to seeing it was so vastly different than my experience of recording it. The emotions didn't match at all, causing a delayed recognition in my mind. I didn't remember it as the perfect, beautiful, carefree moment it appeared to be but as a nice fifteen-second break in the middle of one of my hardest days in recent memory.

We all do this constantly. We apply a dark, grainy, negative filter to everything that comes from our own lives because we know the backstory to every moment. We know that nothing we've experienced felt as good as it looked on the outside.

Because we don't know this about the lives of others, we take their experiences at face value. We assume the moments we have access to felt as good as they looked. We find so little in our own lives that can measure up, and we conclude that our own lives are simply not very good. We spend our days wishing that we could feel the way other people's experiences look, and this mental glitch is the root of all dysfunctional envy.

Luckily, it can be undone.

When you catch yourself getting caught up in debilitating patterns of envy, there are four things I want you to do in order: celebrate, identify, locate, and (sometimes) pursue your desired feeling.

Celebrate

Envy and genuine joy for another person mostly cancel each other out. That's why I want to start by throwing a little celebration for the person you're feeling jealous of. The basis of feelings of envy is that something about the current situation is problematic, wrong, or unfair. Celebrating for the person who has what you want completely changes your mental and emotional framework around the situation. I know this seems absurdly simple, maybe even a little fake or counterintuitive, but please try this technique before writing it off. Every time I use this strategy, I'm reminded of how effective it is.

Many of my therapy clients are much more successful than me in one way or another. When I was newer at providing therapy, and still very much digging myself out of my own hole in life, I had trouble holding empathy for my more high-achieving clients. I couldn't help but feel that I'd be perfectly content with my personal situation if I had what they had, and it's very difficult (impossible, really) to be an effective therapist for someone if you can't hold empathy for them. I found that when I celebrated their wins with them instead of wishing I had what they had, my feelings of envy and jealousy would melt away almost entirely.

It won't always work right away. Sometimes your first reaction when you attempt to be happy for someone else will be a very cynical and snarky response. The words may be right, but the tone is wrong. Your inner dialogue may be sarcastic rather than genuine, like the mental version of a disingenuous slow clapping and a rolling of the eyes. You can probably hear an example of this in your mind right now. It might sound something like *Oooh, yes, I am just* so *happy for them and their perfect life because I know they worked* sooo *hard to get it.* Someone probably reacted to you once (or more than once) in this way and the habit just stuck.

Try not to let yourself get discouraged when this happens. Changing thought patterns and habits is simply a matter of being relentlessly consistent. Your mind has been conditioned to see your fellow humans as competition. We still operate from that resource-scarcity mindset. It may take several repetitions of internally celebrating another person before you're able to feel a genuine sense of happiness or joy for them. It can help to mentally repeat your thoughts like a mantra. The habit of celebrating, rather than envying, other people is developed in the same way the pattern of envy came to be: practice.

Someone you know made three million dollars trading crypto this year? Good! That's freaking awesome for them, and it will probably help them achieve their goals. You see someone who basically has your dream body? Fantastic! They must have sacrificed a lot in life to maintain that. The family across the room in the restaurant you're dining at has three children who are all happily consuming their meals while your lone child is throwing a screaming fit because his chicken tenders have a suboptimal meat-to-breading ratio? Acceptable! (I can't completely put a positive spin on this one because it's a pain I know all too well.) That moment would be even worse if their kids were crying, too.

The world would be an unbelievably terrible place if nobody had special, wonderful things in their lives. Look at what happens in places where people have next to nothing. Theft, assault, and worse can be a part of daily life. In nearly all cases, a positive in someone else's life is a net positive for humanity, and it's not a negative for you specifically. We all need to have sources of joy and contentment in our lives, but none of us gets to have all of them.

It may also help to remember that most of what you want out of life isn't a zero-sum game. In other words, someone else having what you want does not prevent you from also having it or even decrease the likelihood of you having it, unless it's something truly unique, like a specific person being your partner. That smiling mother with the beautiful, content newborn didn't steal her baby from you. The presence of the jacked guy on Instagram with the six-pack does not prevent you from also having a six-pack.

The comedian Jimmy Carr has a very unfunny yet very important quote: "Everybody is jealous of what you've got, but nobody is jealous of how you got it." Unless you're spending large chunks of your day doing literally nothing, the idea that you can add anything to your life is a myth. Every seeming addition is actually a trade where you give up one thing to get something else in return. Anybody who has something you want gave up something to get it. What they gave up may be something you aren't willing to give up. It's important to remember that everything has a cost and not everything is worth the asking price.

Defuse your envy and celebrate the person you feel jealous of by asking and answering the question: *Why is it actually good that this person has what they have?*

Identify

The source of your envy is never what it appears to be. Once you've tempered the initial intensity of the emotion by celebrating the victory of the person you were feeling envious towards, you need to identify the emotional void you were feeling a need to fill. We don't typically feel jealousy towards people unless we aren't feeling very good about the part of our lives we were comparing to theirs. Your envy comes from a sense of longing, a perception of a missing experience where you believe there should be a stronger, more present emotion. We need to correctly identify what that emotion is.

We use achievements and status as a proxy for the feelings we want to experience. In other words, you don't want what the other person has; you want to feel how you think they must feel because of what they have. The possession, achievement, or status is a stand-in for a deeper need. Identifying the missing feeling rather than the missing experience is critical because, while the experience itself may be difficult or even impossible for you to achieve, the feeling you've associated with it is likely obtainable. In fact, you may already have it.

Perhaps you find yourself feeling envious of a YouTuber with a million subscribers. The thought of that many people valuing what they have to say makes you think that they must feel tremendously respected. Respect isn't an emotion you've felt much of recently, so you find yourself wishing you had a popular channel so that you, too, could feel respected.

Or maybe you find yourself feeling envious of someone who appears to have quite a bit of money. You assume that a person with significant financial reserves must feel a great deal of peace in life knowing that they could withstand a disruption in cash flow or a major unexpected expense without much trouble. You haven't experienced a sustained sense of peace in quite some time as your recent years have been fraught with uncertainty, both financial and otherwise, so you find yourself wishing you had more money in order to experience an enduring sense of peace.

Notice how in each of these examples it's actually an emotional experience that we're longing for rather than a possession or a status. We tend to take our thoughts and desires at face value rather than looking at what lies beneath them. This tricks us into thinking the only path to resolution is changing our circumstances. Thankfully it isn't, because the circumstances we find ourselves wanting to change often require years of hard work at best, and they are impossible to achieve at worst.

Everything external that you crave is a middleman to an emotional experience you desire to have more of. In some cases, we can cut out the middleman and find better, more efficient ways to meet our needs. Meeting the need is the purpose of the next section, but don't skip over the part about taking the time to accurately identify the need, or you won't know where to go next.

Identify the feeling missing from your own life that you've artificially connected to the source of your envy by asking and answering the question: *What is it that I believe I would feel if I had this thing I'm longing for?*

Locate

The feeling you're craving may be hiding in plain sight. Once you've identified the absent emotion that caused you to feel envious, make sure it's truly missing from your life and not simply going unnoticed. Our minds respond very strongly to newness and novelty, but they quickly and easily forget about the value of what we already have. You may have untapped sources of the feeling you're longing for in your life already, but you might not be accessing them often enough to experience that emotion consistently.

My wife introduced me to a new concept a few years back called "shopping your home." If you aren't familiar, it means that before impulse buying something, you should look through your home and make sure you don't already own something that can serve the same purpose. Sometimes we throw a new blanket in our online cart on a cold winter day while forgetting about the three perfectly nice blankets neatly folded in the storage chest one room over.

We do this with everything in life, not just material possessions. We spend so much of our lives seeking out redundant emotional experiences that we already have access to. We are black holes of desire, and we inherently want more of whatever is good in our lives. Every pleasant emotion is internally rewarding and therefore at least a little bit addicting. We constantly strive for more life, more respect, more peace, more joy, and more excitement, without stopping to consider if we already have enough.

Before you go chasing a desire sparked by envy, I want you to shop the home of your life. I want you to look at what you already have and see if you're actually missing what seems to be absent. Let me walk you through an example of how to do this.

I was listening to a podcast recently where the guest was a therapist who had opened her own private practice two years ago. She claimed that the practice already had fifty clinicians and was making over a million dollars per year in profit. My practice, a year old at the time, was nowhere near those metrics. Instantly, I felt the familiar pain of envy. Why was she so much better at this than me? My business, which I was feeling decent about five minutes ago, now seemed pathetic in comparison.

I took a moment to turn my attention away from the podcast and instead look inward, reflecting on my emotional state. There were a few feelings swirling around inside my mind, but one stood out above the rest: I felt incompetent. Listening to that podcast had convinced me that I had no idea what I was doing as a business owner. In all fairness, it's not terribly hard to convince me of such things given that I'm a chronically insecure individual with an avoidant/dismissive attachment style. If you aren't familiar with attachment styles, us avoidant/dismissives are the ones who keep people well outside the boundaries of our hearts due to our massive insecurities about everything because people didn't hug us enough when we were small.

This look inward gave me the information I needed. I was feeling a lack of competence, a deficit of proof that I was a reasonably skilled human being who is good at some things. I didn't need to scale my practice to ten times the size it was at the time, which was great news, because even after finishing the podcast I still had no idea how I was supposed to do that. I just needed to find some reasons to feel competent in that moment, whether in business or otherwise. I asked another question inwardly: *OK brain, what are we really good at?*

Answering that question helped remind me that I have plenty of reasons to feel competent. I'm a decent cook (especially if charcoal is involved); I can catch a fish on just about any body of water; I think I'm a pretty good therapist; my tree identification skills are on point; and my hygiene is excellent. I'm good at many things that matter quite a bit to me. Whether the world values these things or not may be a different story, but my brain, my emotions. That's my rule and it applies to you, too. It would be great to have a million-dollar business, but the absence of that does not make me incompetent.

Put another way, "We already have feelings of competence at home."

The goal here is not to pursue the shallow parts of someone else's life but the deep parts of your own. You want to scan your life for every possible source of that emotion and work to fully mine each vein of that feeling. So often, our appreciation of the special things in our lives is shallow. Our minds do this automatically, and it takes conscious effort to practice full appreciation of what we already have, which is often the final nail in the coffin of maladaptive feelings of envy.

Locate and tap into already available sources of the missing feeling by asking and answering the question: *What sources of this feeling already exist in my life, and how I can access them right now?*

Pursue

Sometimes there's a fourth step in this process. Once you've practiced your paradoxical celebration, identified what feeling was missing inside of you, and found already available ways for you to access that feeling, you'll end up with one of two outcomes: You'll either feel reasonably content with your life and a bit silly for spiraling over missing something you already had, or you'll find that some genuine desire for change remains. Sometimes there is a kernel of truth in our jealous longings, an actual lifestyle problem that needs to be addressed.

To continue with my example from the last section, after noticing jealousy over someone else's financial situation and celebrating their success, realizing I was correlating their financial success with a feeling of competency, and identifying and accessing sources of competency that already existed in my own life, I may still be left with a genuine desire to improve my financial health. This doesn't mean I failed to manage my feelings of envy. Quite the opposite; I have now transformed my envy into a behavioral goal.

Paradoxically, envy tends to hold us back from making real change and accomplishing our goals. The strong, overwhelming sense of jealousy that hits in our initial moment of longing usually carries with it a false sense of urgency, even panic, that causes us to move towards the object of our desires in fits and starts rather than with sustained, consistent effort. This usually causes us to get frustrated and, eventually, quit working on our goals altogether.

When we break free of the frantic dysfunctional drive of envy, we're often left with a healthy, adaptive striving for something desirable. Our thought process becomes less *I suck and I'm a worthless person until I achieve this* and more *I think I would enjoy being me more if I was able to accomplish this.*

If you unearth a legitimate desire to improve something in your life once your envy has been washed away, you should pursue that desire. None of us are out here living perfect lives, and moving towards goals that are not driven by dysfunctional emotions almost always produces positive outcomes in the contexts of quality of life and overall mental health.

Determine if and how you want to pursue the goal that remains after the envy has been stripped away by asking and answering the question: *Do I still feel a need to improve this area of my life even after accessing my missing feeling, and if so, how should I improve it?*

My second lesson to you is this: Every experience of envy is born of ignorance about what it's actually like to be anybody except yourself.

If all else fails, remember: It's just potatoes.

Truth Three

Don't Let the Darkness In

The Story

The Forest

The forest surrounding the lake was unfathomably vast and dense. Mostly evergreens, a roughly equal mix of pine, spruce, and fir, with occasional birches, maples, and oaks thrown in for variety, the line of trees seemed to stretch on forever. On a satellite map, it looked like a massive green ocean dotted with the occasional blue island of a lake. The trunks of the trees were so close together you couldn't see more than fifteen or twenty feet in before everything looked black. It was a stunning drive, especially in the fall when hues of yellow, orange, and red broke up the vibrant green expanse.

There was a particular grove of trees in our side yard that I loved. It was filled with red pine trees, and a lone massive oak sat in the center. Red pine trees have a very odd and distinct growth pattern: All of their lower limbs fall off as they grow. They can reach heights of over one hundred feet, but only the highest ten to fifteen feet have any branches, giving them the appearance of a flagpole with a tree on top. Some of my happiest childhood memories are simply lying on my back in the grove and staring up at the spot where the sunlight could be seen between the leaves.

The only major road in the area weaved its way through the sparsest sections of timber, the branches stretching out from the shoulder, nearly scraping the windows of passing cars. Every few miles, small trails split off from the main road. You can barely see them unless you know where to look. It's a total inversion of the typical relationship between humans and nature. Here, people are the minority, the obligatory little blips on a wild, mostly untamed radar.

You could spend your entire life here and barely see a fraction of all it has to offer. With over half a million acres of forest and easily more than a thousand lakes, many of which don't have a single house on them, the recreational opportunities are functionally limitless. There is more here than a single human could ever know, and it's always changing.

Having spent so much of my childhood in the forest, I sometimes forget how jarring a place like this can be for those who didn't grow up here. In our twenties, my wife and I brought two other couples on vacation with us here, each in our own vehicle, and as we drove farther into the forest, the nervousness in their text messages was apparent.

"Are we lost?"

"How the heck did you guys find this place?"

"Do . . . people really live here?"

The first morning, one of them went outside of the cabin to relieve himself, as the only bathroom was in use, only to quickly return and voice his intent to never go outside again after seeing "the biggest, most terrifying bug in existence." I glanced outside to see a hummingbird flit by the window. For the remainder of the trip, hummingbirds were referred to as "terrordactyls."

Growing up surrounded by the forest, I assumed that it had been there since the beginning of time. I had never seen such an ancient-looking place. Some of the white pines towered over one hundred feet tall. Standing underneath of them and staring up to the sky provided a dizzying sense of scale.

The ecosystem contained an entire food chain spanning from gnats to timber wolves and black bears. You never knew what you might spot if you peered deeply enough between the trees. There was a truly incomprehensible amount of wildlife under the forest canopy.

Despite its ancient appearance, the forest was barely one hundred years old when I was first introduced to it. If we had visited this area around the turn of the twentieth century, we would have seen nothing but barren, empty land. The ecosystem in this area was almost completely annihilated by an all-too-common mix of ignorance, callousness, and greed. A destructive power had forced its way into this region and torn down tremendous quantities of organic life.

This massive forest wasn't some archaic region predating humanity; it was the rebirth of an area devastated by an unimaginable trauma. It was a symbol of resilience and recovery, not of invincible endurance. I had a very difficult time accepting that something so massive and strong could simultaneously be so vulnerable and wounded, but the lore of the forest's rebirth was well documented.

In the early to mid-1800s, logging companies began to move into the Midwest. A massive population boom had created an unanticipated need for hardwood for building new homes. Many of the forests along the East Coast had been stripped bare by the operational practices of these massive corporations. Wood was also the primary source of energy at that time, the internal combustion engine having not been invented yet, and the need for natural resources was at an all-time high.

The word "conservation" had yet to be introduced to the corporate vocabulary. The logging companies were allowed to operate unrestricted in this area, and they completely stripped it down to grass and bare earth. Scores of lumberjacks came to the forest with saws and wagons and the intent of removing as much lumber as possible from the region, and they were highly successful at doing so.

Their only concern was profit. Millions of acres of natural habit were destroyed. Countless animals perished, suddenly lacking the food and shelter needed to survive, as their former homes were burned in the furnace of industry. Death and destruction trailed in humanity's wake as it swept across the forest.

The lumberjacks themselves got little out of the deal. Most lived in lice-infested group bunks, worked fourteen-hour days, ate gruel, and spent the majority of their meager paychecks on alcohol at the nearest local bar. Brawls were constant, injuries common, and gruesome deaths a regular occurrence. There were few harder lots in life. Only those atop the corporate hierarchy saw any benefit from the reaping of the woods.

Nearly all the forested areas in the Midwest were logged barren during this time. The few that weren't were instead burned through by forest fires sparked by human carelessness. Fire safety wasn't really a concept yet either, with Smokey Bear's critical warnings coming about fifty years later. Respecting organic life was not on anybody's radar.

The world took what it wanted from this region and left it a barren wasteland. The forest was sacrificed to the endless churning of the "progress" machine. No humans lived here so nobody cared. The lumberjacks only stayed in their camps as long as there was work here, then they packed up and moved on to the next area.

When the logging was complete, the only remaining traces of the trees were the seeds buried beneath the soil. The forest must have looked completely dead to the naked eye, with the only surviving remnants of what once thrived now hidden away from the world. It was in the throes of death without a doubt, but the seeds offered one last source of hope. If they could sprout into trees, the forest might be able to regenerate.

The land needed protection and time to heal. Thankfully it was given that. This area was one of the first designated national forests in the United States. Someone recognized that, with appropriate assistance, something wonderful could regrow here. Boundaries were defined and rules were created. This area was never to be logged again.

It seems impossible that anything so thoroughly devastated as this forest could ever grow back into what it once was. Millions of acres of timber were removed in our county alone. But incredibly, with time and care, something beautiful and vibrant began to emerge.

Experiencing the forest's gradual regrowth must have been awe inspiring. Many of the trees that were taken down were hundreds of years old. A completely new ecosystem was created when they were first logged, as the region morphed from a forest to a plain. With no leaf canopy to create shade, wild grasses and plants were briefly able to thrive with minimal competition.

Before long, saplings sprouted across the plains. The tiny trees were fragile yet optimistic signs of recovery, the next phase of the seeds once forgotten under the soil. Though capable of growing into something powerful and resilient, they were still quite vulnerable at this stage. Many were eaten by wildlife or outcompeted for sunlight and water by other plants.

With each passing year, the surviving saplings grew taller and stronger. Eventually, they stood well above the bushes and shrubs, establishing themselves as the harbingers of a new beginning. They were more resilient now, threatened only by extreme weather conditions. Slowly but surely, the rebirth of over half a million acres of destruction was well underway.

Eventually, the plains looked like a forest again. Not a forest full of white pines towering hundreds of feet tall, as it once was, but a forest teeming with birds, thriving with deer, and smelling like leaves and wood, nonetheless. This is the version of the forest I met as a child.

Even after over a hundred years of recovery, the forest is not fully healed yet. I know this because I've seen into the past, in my own way. There's a small section of the forest that was never logged due to a mapping error. It was mistakenly indicated as a lake instead of timber, so the lumberjacks worked around it rather than through it. This place has remained untouched since the beginning of creation.

When you enter this lost area, you can instantly see the difference between a hundred-year-old forest and a thousand-year-old forest. The most mature trees here are far older than any living person and taller than most buildings. The huge white pines that tower over the maples and the oaks in the main forest look juvenile by comparison. The tree canopy is so far above the ground that it seems to reach the clouds and so dense that the forest floor is nothing but dirt in most places. The lost area is ancient, a place forgotten by time.

The air is different here, like the contrast between tap water and filtered water. You can taste a crispness on your tongue, an organic and pure sensation that fills your lungs with energy and life. With billions of leaves and virtually no pollution to filter, there is an organicity to the air that I'd love to bottle up and turn into a cologne. It would be a best seller for sure.

The quiet calm is almost eerie, especially if you aren't used to being in such a place. It's one of the only spaces I've entered that has no hint of human control. You always feel like a visitor here, although not an unwelcome one.

The lost area offers a vision of the past but also an image of a potential future. At just over a hundred years into its journey of rebirth, the forest is thriving again, but it hasn't fully recovered. The trauma, damage, and destruction caused by an uncaring world was tremendous. It will take at least another century for the woods to fully grow back, but they have everything they need to recover. The only missing piece is time.

Very broadly speaking, there are three categories of restrictions people who enter the forest must abide by:

- No living thing inside of the forest can be damaged or destroyed. Obviously this prohibits logging, but even something as simple as picking a mushroom or a flower is forbidden.
- Nothing potentially dangerous to the environment can be brought into the forest. You cannot bring fireworks, lighter fluid, or toxic chemicals into this region.
- No inorganic materials are to be left inside of the forest. Anything you enter with you must leave with. Don't leave your trash in the forest.

The forest could never have recovered without help. It required boundaries, rules, and protections to create the conditions that allowed for the regrowth that it needed. When those supports are present, nearly any damage can be healed in time.

The Lesson

Regrowth

Living things can recover from almost anything if they are properly protected from further damage and given space and time to regrow. This was very good news for me, as I had quite a bit to recover from.

Although I don't think my mind was ever "healthy," I was a very different person for the first twelve years of my life than I was for the following ten. Something began to change inside of me, stripping away what little organic love, peace, and joy had grown, and leaving me barren and burned inside. Any remnants of the kind, inquisitive, adventurous boy were buried underneath years of pain and rejection.

Not only did I make no effort to halt this transformation, I actively encouraged it. It seemed inevitable, desirable even, that I would become something else. I wasn't literally trying to kill myself during this period of my life, but I think I was trying to kill the boy within, the sensitive, fragile soul that the world didn't seem to value.

I always had the sense that something was different about me, "off" in some intangible way. Even early on in life when I had a relatively large friend group, it somehow always felt like I was on the outside of the circle looking in. I used to wonder if I was truly human or if I was something else. Maybe I was a robot, programmed to blend in with humanity but lacking a few necessary lines of code. Or perhaps I was an alien sent to Earth as a spy to gather data for a future intergalactic war.

The social challenges that come with adolescence are hard for nearly everyone to adapt to, but I seemed to be even more ill prepared for them than most. It felt like I missed the starting gun for a race I didn't even know I was supposed to be running. By the time I looked up, everyone was already several miles down the road, and I was all alone.

I was generally well-liked in elementary school, but once middle school started, it seemed like I was trying to hold on to parts of my childhood that everyone else had readily abandoned. I desperately wanted another year or two of recess and games and exploring never-ending green forests. My peers could tell that I wasn't maturing at the same rate as they were, which resulted in a lot of teasing and bullying about my speech, my clothing, and my hobbies. This world can be particularly cruel to those who move at their own organic pace, and struggle with, or simply resist, the course of life that comes naturally to most people.

Because I hadn't faced rejection on a scale like this before, I had no plan for it. In a desperate, panicked attempt to stop the social bleeding, I did whatever the people who seemed to be well-liked and respected told me to do. I thought that if I let the norms and values of others into my inner space, erasing my thoughts and feelings and overriding them with whatever these people had inside of them, I might be more successful at conforming to the world's expectations of me.

My rationale for this plan was that those who were going at the "correct" pace in life must have some secret wisdom or knowledge that had been withheld from me. Perhaps if I spent enough time with them and observed their habits I could learn how to fit in. I became an adolescent anthropologist in reverse, a chimp studying Jane Goodall in a desperate attempt to learn how to pass for human.

For the most part, I let anyone else do whatever they wanted to me without resistance. I wouldn't argue with even the most hurtful of insults that were thrown at me, thinking that if I rolled with the punches, I might change their minds about whether I was worthy of companionship. Some of my "friends" were physically aggressive to me at times, and I made no attempt to stop them. I allowed people to steal from me, thinking that they might have more positive associations with me if they enjoyed some of my former possessions.

Some of the things I allowed people to do to me were bad enough that I won't write about them here, in order to keep this book as trauma friendly as possible. Despite hating every second of it, allowing people to treat me however they pleased seemed like the only way out of the hole I had fallen into. If being me didn't work, I would simply try being whatever others wanted me to be. If the world couldn't value me as a person, perhaps it could find value in me as a resource to be consumed.

I also tried to make myself like whatever the people I looked up to happened to like. My hobbies, interests, and even choices in things like music and television shows conformed and regressed to the average of my social circle. Anything that made me stand out made me a target and therefore had to be eliminated at all costs. No weaknesses or openings could be left. "Different" became a synonym for "vulnerable," and anything unique about me was like a tree sticking out above the forest canopy: far too visible and in need of immediate removal.

My only criteria for letting someone into my life was that they had to be a person who showed interest in me. They didn't even have to act like they liked me. They just had to acknowledge me and pay attention to me in literally any way. That's how desperate I was for peer socialization and approval. There was no dare too ridiculous, too stupid, or too dangerous for me to accept in the pursuit of a potential increase in social status.

There's a cognitive distortion, or thinking error, called the "just world fallacy." The premise is that when we (falsely) believe the world is a fair and righteous place, we assume that whatever we get from the world is what we deserve. If people hurt us, we deserve to be hurt. If people insult us, we deserve to be insulted. Every negative experience is an appropriate and reasonable reaction to something that's wrong with us. We can be treated better by becoming better.

Although I wasn't aware of the concept at the time, I thoroughly bought into the just world fallacy. I started to assume that the way the people in my life treated me reflected the way I deserved to be treated. I assumed that if I was worthy of love, people would love me. It never occurred to me that perhaps the people I was surrounding myself with simply weren't the right people for me. I remember being told repeatedly that I could do anything and be anything, and at that point in my life the only thing I wanted to be was like everybody else. I was willing to do whatever it took to make that happen.

Despite my best efforts, none of these dramatic life changes improved my social situation to any noticeable degree. I think people can tell when they're interacting with a persona rather than a person, and the way I was acting was anything but natural to me. The inorganic nature of my interactions with others just made me come across as even more awkward than before.

When it became clear that my planned, intentional conformity strategy wasn't ever going to work, I gave up on it entirely. It required immense effort and provided me with absolutely nothing in return. The transformation never felt complete. There was still too much of me inside. I had planted the correct seeds to make myself like everyone else, but I don't think I ever had the right soil.

Once I accepted that I could not be like them and would never be liked by them, I decided to try a different approach. If I couldn't form relationships with other people, maybe I could connect with the darkness itself. Despite not really fitting in, the hate, shame, and callousness around me had started to become a part of me, like toxic chemicals seeping into the soil after a spill.

I desperately wanted to be the best at something, but I didn't feel like I was particularly good at anything that mattered. There was only one part of my life where I thought I might have an edge over anyone I knew: I could be the most damaged, unhinged, and unpredictable person in the world. Being remarkably broken seemed somehow preferrable to being thoroughly unremarkable.

I nurtured the darkness inside of me and fought to suppress the light. My ability to care about other people disappeared almost entirely, other than in ways that were very self-serving. I began to see women as objects of desire instead of living human beings worthy of respect. Other people were nothing more than vehicles that could be used to reach certain emotional destinations. Momentary pleasure, power, and status became the only meaningful pursuits. There was no hope of having anything else.

Parallel to this goal was a desire to remove myself from humanity without dying. I thought that if I stopped loving or caring about anything and found a way to destroy my emotions, nothing would ever hurt again. Emotional anesthesia seemed preferrable to chronic pain. This would necessitate scrubbing my backstory from existence, so I set about doing just that. I instructed my parents to take down every childhood photo of me and put it into storage. They were clearly disturbed by the request, but they complied, presumably and understandably having no clue what to do with me at this point. Who has a game plan for what to do if your child doesn't want to be human anymore?

If something could change how I thought or felt, I would gladly put it into my body. The only limits were access and quantity. I would do more of whatever I had than anyone else around me, to demonstrate the power of my brokenness. My emotions and behaviors were unpredictable and irrational, and those around me became just as afraid of my mind as I was.

I could feel the person I used to be slipping away as I intentionally exposed myself to the worst the world had to offer. Seeking out the most depressing, rage-filled music amplified the sadness and the anger already inside of me. Watching the most violent, disturbing movies and TV shows made me hate humanity even more, which made it easier to distance myself from it. I wore my brokenness like a general's uniform, each trauma a unique medal of honor.

By surrounding myself with the anarchistic, the misanthropic, the rejected, and the lost, I had finally found my people. I aligned heavily with the beliefs and values of the goth and punk subcultures and fell into all the behaviors that, at least in my region, were characteristic of people who held those values. Drug use. Massive relational drama (even by teenage standards). Mayhem. Vandalism and destruction of property. Self-harm. We seemed to alternate between taking our anger out on ourselves and taking it out on others.

After years of loneliness and isolation, I had located the dark little corner of the world where I belonged. In this part of the world, I could have value. The group I was part of now seemed to understand my pain. They hated the world with me instead of hating me with the world.

Plan A, conforming to the world while granting it unlimited access to me, had failed spectacularly, but Plan B, embracing the chaos and the destruction, was working seamlessly. The boy inside of me was dying rapidly, and in his place something much darker was growing. I began to make plans to do terrible things to this world that was so terrible to me.

But something in the forest saved me.

The summer after I finished high school, my parents convinced me to take a trip with just them up north. To this day I don't know if they realized how close I was to not being here anymore or if the timing of the trip was pure coincidence. There wasn't much of me left to connect with, as my skills for typical social interactions had decayed so badly that I could barely hold a normal conversation.

I'm not sure exactly why I agreed to take a trip that was entirely counterproductive to my goals at the time. My grudging acceptance was very conditional; I kept my headphones on for the duration of the drive, only spoke when I felt like it (which was almost never), and demanded solitude and privacy whenever I felt like withdrawing. They granted me this without hesitation.

Most of the drive was uneventful, but as we ventured farther north and entered the forest from my childhood, I became aware of something buried deep inside of me. At first, I was certain that it was my imagination, memories of feelings I could no longer access. The farther into the forest we went the more undeniable it became. The boy wasn't dead after all.

Every outward expression of hope, desire, and love had been chopped down and burned away, but the seeds of these feelings had survived somehow. They were dry, dormant, and entirely lacking in nutrients, but they had remained under the soil for years, waiting for the right conditions to start growing again.

I had tried so hard to erase my relatively happy memories and the connections I had formed with people. I believed they were nothing more than a liability preventing me from embracing the shadow version of myself I needed to become to win the respect and approval of the world. I had failed. Thank God I had failed. It was only among the trees that I could finally admit it. This was never what I wanted but what I thought I had to settle for. What I really wanted was my old life and feelings back. I wanted to go back to the fork in the road and take the other path this time. My conformity to the social patterns of this world was not rooted in a genuine desire. It was nothing more than the fawn response of an abuse victim.

We spent about a week there, and with every day my conviction grew. Seeing the forest reminded me that, once, something equally beautiful was thriving within me before I encouraged the darkness of the world to consume it. It provided me with all the proof I needed that a rebirth is possible even if the magnitude of the destruction is tremendous. There was still something inside of me worth protecting and preserving. Maybe with enough time and care it, too, could heal, just like the forest did.

When we came back from that trip, something different was growing inside of me. Though my regeneration was far from complete, I had found just enough goodness left to nurture. The journey back to the forest wasn't the moment when everything changed and nothing hurt anymore. Twenty-five years later, I am still reclaiming pieces of my heart from the darkness that tried to steal it. But it was that moment when I realized my mistake and corrected my course.

Going forward, there would be rules about who and what was allowed to enter my life. No more unrestricted access to my mind or my body. No more polluting my mind with ideas of what I was instructed to like by those who didn't understand me or care about me. Nothing would enter my space that didn't interact well with what was already growing there.

And if there wasn't a place in this world where a person like me belonged, I would be the one to create it.

The Application

Scrutinize the Lies

There is a darkness in this world that wants to make its way inside of you. I'm sure you've felt its call. It has a particular knack for finding people like us. The ones whose souls can't seem to find a home in this world. The forgotten. The lost. The abandoned. Our most painful emotions are like gaping wounds that allow the polluted fog to seep inside of us.

It preys on sadness, rejection, and isolation. It grows in the shadows of insecurity, failure, and shame. With enough sunlight and water, it becomes a monster inside of you, a force of hatred and revenge claiming to be an avenging angel willing to right the wrongs the world has inflicted on you. By rewarding and reinforcing the most painful parts of your experience and the most shameful parts of your identity, it pulls you even further away from the hope and the answers you long for.

It promises everything you've ever wanted, yet everything it promises is a lie. You have to be able to scrutinize the lies if you hope to resist its call. Some of its guarantees are simply empty and hollow, debts you will never be able to collect on. Others will be given to you, but in a way that leaves you ruined and broken inside. Just like I was.

The darkness has many names. Some call it the devil. Some call it the heart of man. Some call it society. Whatever title you choose to give it doesn't alter the reality of what we're all up against. Evil exists and it is oddly infectious.

Do not let it in. There are things inside of you that are worth preserving. So many wonderful things. They still live within you today even if you haven't felt their presence in ages. They can never be fully taken from you.

I'm very aware that you've been taught otherwise time and time again. So many of your experiences up to this point have sown and nurtured the seeds of self-hatred. The adversity you've faced from nearly every direction has forced your organic self deeper and deeper inside of you, hidden as far away as possible from the axes, saws, and matches of society. This world may not have treated you as something with tremendous value, but the world isn't always right.

The darkness promises you that you'll have the love of the world, or at least the section of it that you value, if you simply conform and obey. This is a lie. It's impossible to be loved by the world as the world itself does not love. True love is a feeling you will only receive from a few people, at most, over the course of your life. There simply isn't enough time in this life for more than a handful of humans to know you well enough to truly feel love for you.

Tragically, these unique, special people who are capable of loving us are so often the ones we leave behind in our pursuit of global appreciation and admiration. The darkness inside of us tells us that it's not enough, that we need more. Much more. It reassures us that the pain inside will finally go away if we secure enough goodwill from enough people. When we act on these reassurances, we risk losing what little genuine connection can be found in this life. If the love of one, two, or three people cannot satisfy you, the number you're likely to end up with instead is zero.

The darkness swears that you'll have what you've always wanted if you just do what it tells you. Your goals will be met, your dreams finally realized. These misleading promises are customized for each of us, connected to our deepest fantasies. For some of us they will involve power and influence, others beauty and strength, and others still wealth and riches.

This lie is particularly deceptive, because if you're willing to use, abuse, and manipulate people, you may indeed get what you want on the surface, but these accomplishments will leave you feeling hollow and empty inside. What you really want is to feel the way you believe you would feel if you accomplished those goals, and aligning with the darkness weakens your ability to feel anything in the light. You can have everything yet feel nothing, as so many do.

Resisting this darkness is a battle you must fight every day no matter how strong you are. It will feel utterly impossible at times. Most people give in for at least a while. Many give in forever. When you resist, you'll be living with a constant awareness that you're swimming against the tide. You won't feel "normal."

Worse, sometimes it won't even feel like a battle. When there is already darkness inside of you, it feels perfectly natural to soak in the darkness outside of you. There is a sense of alignment, compatibility. This is exactly how I felt. It was as if I had finally found the ally who shared the immense anger and pain that always seemed to follow me.

If you've already let these things into your heart, please know that it isn't too late for you. That was one of my biggest mistakes, thinking that I had crossed some imagined point of no return. It took a chance visual reminder of something so much bigger and greater than me to convince me that I wasn't permanently broken and hopelessly lost. Regrowth is always possible, but it may require dramatic change.

What needs to change most are the permissions you've set for who and what is allowed access to your inner self. To resist the darkness of this world, you need to have boundaries: boundaries with people, boundaries with media consumption, and boundaries with yourself and the thoughts, feelings, and behaviors you feed and grow inside of you. Just as there are rules for entering a national forest, there must also be rules for letting things and people enter your life if you wish to preserve everything natural and organic inside.

Every environment is shaped by access and restrictions. Controlling who and what is allowed to enter a space determines whether it can remain organic and natural, or whether it slowly conforms to the spreading development surrounding it. If you let anyone into your mind and your heart who desires access, eventually your thoughts and feelings become the mental equivalent of one of those neighborhoods that's just row after row of identical houses. We celebrate visible diversity in many ways, but we seem to have trouble respecting mental diversity.

Not everyone deserves to have access to you. Everything that you allow to enter your inner environment becomes a part of you. Your relationships, even those that are shorter and less intense, will permanently leave you with little parts of the other person inside of you well after the relationships run their course. Some of these parts will be like light and water and fertilizer to everything inside of you: They will support a stronger, healthier growth of what was already there. Other parts will be like herbicide, killing anything organic they encounter and leaving barren, damaged spots within.

Relationships with other people are arguably the strongest influence that pushes our lives in one direction or another. They certainly were for me. The people in your life fundamentally change your beliefs, habits, interests, and personality traits. You become the statistical average of your immediate peer group. You will think like them, feel like them, live like them, and see the world as they see it.

Some people will enter your inner world in a kind and respectful manner. They will take care not to damage or destroy what you allow them to access. They tread carefully and lightly, making sure not to leave anything behind that belongs to them and not to you. That doesn't mean that these people will never ask you to change or challenge you to grow, but when they do, it will come from a place of love and honor rather than jealousy or callousness. They simply want you to be the best possible version of you and seek to nurture and strengthen what's already inside of you rather than to remove it and plant something more appealing to them.

Other people will blast into your inner world in a lifted truck, windows down and music blaring, doing donuts in your ecosystem and throwing their empty beer cans out the window. I myself drive a lifted truck, so I am allowed to stereotype here. These people don't come into your life with the intention of damaging you, but they certainly won't be careful to avoid it. They simply lack the ability to appreciate the beauty of the space that they've entered, so they take no care to honor it. If you let them in, they will almost certainly damage you with their carelessness.

A third category of person enters your life methodically with axes, saws, and a coherent plan. They want to destroy the goodness inside of you. Maybe they're jealous of what you have, but since they cannot find a way to acquire it for themselves, they've decided the next best way to even the score is to make sure you don't have it either. Perhaps they're so fully given over to their own inner darkness that they cannot bear to see anything standing in defiance of it and feel a pull to destroy it. Regardless of their rationale, these people mean you direct and intentional harm and should be kept out at all costs.

The media we choose to expose ourselves to also reshapes our inner environments. We usually seek out songs, shows, and influencers that strengthen and reinforce what's already inside of us. If we're generally angry, we usually like angry music, frustrated people, violent movies, and intense, visceral content. If we mostly feel sadness, we're more drawn to the slow-paced, the melancholy, the disenchanted, and the gray.

It's only natural to seek out validation and confirmation of our feelings, but when our ratio of media choices skews heavily in the direction of painful emotions, we often end up in a self-perpetuating cycle. When most of what we see, hear, and feel reinforces unpleasant feelings, we run the risk of moving things like sadness and anger from acute experiences into core parts of our identities. They become observable personality traits that change how others react to us and what opportunities are available to us, falsely confirming our fears that the things that make us different are inherently maladaptive and problematic.

Feeling sadness won't ruin your life, but identifying with the sadness to such a degree that it's all anyone can see when they look at you certainly can. It's also a massive oversimplification of the complex being you truly are. No matter how large your sadness feels, there's more to you than that. There always has been and there always will be.

Everything you see and hear consistently feels "normal." Our minds use repetition as a proxy for "good" or "healthy" because we're bombarded with so many ideas we can't possibly think critically about each and every one of them. Put a different way, your brain doesn't fully comprehend that you're hate-watching mukbang videos, but it suddenly has an entirely unrelated urge to binge eat nachos grande.

Please be so cautious about what you normalize for yourself with your media choices.

We also can and should have boundaries with the things that originate from inside of us. Not all of your thoughts are winners. Some of your feelings are not based in anything real. Many of your urges and impulses are more than happy to destroy your life if you overindulge in them. Some of these inner experiences need to be taken captive. Others need to be taken out back and disposed of.

Consider evaluating your thoughts on how they correlate with your perception of reality and your goals for the future. No matter how hard you work on yourself and your life, you're always going to have those rogue thoughts that have absolutely nothing to do with anything presently happening in your life. You know the ones. You're at your job minding your own business and trying to get some work done or making dinner for your kids when suddenly your brain informs you that you're a hopeless loser who has never done anything and never will do anything, and you should just end it now.

They're sort of like drive-by insults, devoid of context and completely detached from the current reality. Yet we're so often tempted to indulge them and engage with them because they activate our negativity bias. If they were true they would be terrible, so we consider them and ponder them to make sure that they aren't, and before we know it, we're aligned with them. They need to be evicted from your mind with a simple, authoritative dismissal. Something along the lines of *Nope, stupid thought, next.* That won't magically stop them from happening, but retraining your thought process in this manner is similar to resetting your social media algorithm. With enough time and after many mental instances of clicking "I am not interested in this," the frequency of seeing this content will finally start to go down.

Emotions work very similarly. You can be in the middle of a reasonable pleasant experience and suddenly get hit with crushing sadness or debilitating fear out of absolutely nowhere. Sometimes there will be a thought connected to it. You'll be watching your children or your pets enjoying a pleasant moment when that dark voice in your mind insists upon being heard. *Don't forget that they're going to die someday.* Instantly your enjoyment of the moment is ruined.

Sometimes the emotion isn't connected to anything conscious. The joy, peace, or excitement you were feeling a second ago just disappears for no apparent reason. Sometimes it's replaced with inexplicable loneliness or random dissatisfaction. Other times it's replaced with nothing at all and just leaves the sensation of a gaping hole inside of you.

Regardless of which version of the fickle, fluctuating emotional state you're in, it's important to acknowledge to yourself when your feelings are in direct opposition to your present experience. When you feel sad about nothing, remind yourself that you're currently sad about nothing. That isn't to say that your life is perfect in that moment, and you could certainly find something to be sad about if you tried hard enough, but this is the trap our emotions often lead us into. We have a feeling, we don't know why we have that feeling, so we scan our life for every possible source of that emotion, accidentally ruminating on every problem we're currently facing while doing so. This gives us our "reason" for feeling sad, but there was no initial reason. It was a random emotional impulse that we justified, to no benefit to ourselves, through reasoning.

When considering behaviors or behavioral impulses, I try to regularly ask and answer the question: *What is (or what would be) the purpose of doing this right now?* Sometimes there is a very clear and legitimate answer to that question, such as *I'm going to lie down because I'm not feeling well and I think I need to rest.* Sometimes there's an answer, but I don't like the answer. *I'm picking up my phone and opening Instagram because that's more immediately gratifying than writing another sentence of this book* is not a satisfactory answer to me, therefore I do not act on the impulse. Sometimes there's no reason at all. We make a disturbing number of decisions with absolutely no conscious thought behind them, roughly 80 percent according to some estimates. Consider eliminating as many behaviors as possible that serve no clear purpose in your life..

Every major part of your life should be subject to this level of scrutiny. Nothing should be allowed in and given attention automatically. There needs to be a guard at the door of your heart and your mind, and he needs to be very particular about his criteria. If you don't make conscious, mindful decisions about who and what to let in, your mind will be reshaped without your consent.

You absolutely must place boundaries on who and what is allowed to access you. These boundaries should be based upon your long-term goals for yourself and your vision for your life. I form and maintain my personal boundaries by regularly asking and answering clarifying questions about my life. Here are some of the questions I encourage you to ask and answer in order to keep your inner space healthy and thriving:

Who was I before the darkness took over?

- If there was a point in your life before things started to go downhill, what was different about that period compared to now?
- How did the happiest, healthiest, most functional version of yourself live, think, and feel compared to your current self?
- How could you reintegrate some of the elements of that person's life into your current life?

Who do I wish to become in the future?

- What values do you want to organize your life around?
- What personality traits do you wish you possessed more of?
- What emotions do you wish your life contained more of? How could you access these emotions more consistently?

What would move me closer to becoming this person?

- What is present in the life of this ideal version of yourself that is absent from your life?
- What is absent in the life of this ideal version of yourself that is present in your life?
- How would this person allocate their time differently than you currently do?

What do I understand my purpose in this world to be?

- Do you have any particular skills or gifts that might help other people or the world in general?
- Do you believe that your experience here connects to any greater meaning or purpose?

My third lesson to you is this: Do not let the darkness of this world into your heart. Continue to ask and answer the questions that pull you away from the hate and the negativity of this place, and keep your inner space healthy and thriving. Remember that nothing is too damaged to experience regrowth, or even rebirth under the correct circumstances, and that the person responsible for creating and maintaining these circumstances is you.

Truth Four

Pull the Weeds

The Story

The Flowers

The hardest part of any long trip is the middle. The beginning has optimism, the promise of tremendous adventure waiting for you on the other side of a war of attrition between your excitement and your patience. The end has reward, a tremendous sense of achievement stemming from the long-awaited outcome being almost tangible after enduring for so long. But the middle of the journey lacks either of these.

The middle is where the reality of what you're truly up against sets in. The hope and optimism from the start of the journey have faded, but you aren't close enough to your destination to feel the excitement. You're stuck in this car for quite some time, and it's going to be a while before anything interesting happens. You're trapped inside your mind with nothing but your own thoughts to occupy you, which is a terrifying proposition if you're anything like me.

I always needed entertainment on long road trips. Prior to cell phones I had to rely on books, magazines, puzzles, my Game Boy, and later, a power converter with a tiny television and a PlayStation 1. My parents always thought I got bored easily, which wasn't entirely untrue, but it wasn't the main reason I constantly craved outlets for my attention. I just couldn't stand hearing my own thoughts.

Young me would have been the easiest person in the world to torture. You wouldn't have had to do anything at all to my body. You'd just have to leave me alone in a quiet room with nothing but my own mind to keep me company, and what it would do to me would be far worse than anything you could come up with. I'd tell you all my secrets before the first day was over.

My mind began to ask questions that I had no hope of answering at around age six. Questions like, *What's the point of continuing to live?* or *Why would God love somebody like me?* As far as I could tell, nobody else was thinking about these things, and if they were, they certainly weren't doing it out loud. Everyone else appeared to just exist and function without these concerns weighing them down, so I assumed I was expected to be able to do the same.

Keeping my questions pressed up against the back of my mind where they didn't completely overwhelm me required constant mental effort any time I was bored. My weak and terrified consciousness tried desperately to hold the door shut as an invading army with a battering ram tried to break it down and open me up to another existential crisis. No matter what I had just done, it never took long for the discontentment to surge forth from my subconscious during the quiet times.

Unfortunately, the drive from central Iowa to northern Minnesota is not a terribly exciting one. The vast majority of the space between where we lived and where we vacationed was farmland, and while I love to explore farmland, looking at it from a car window gets old quickly. There's little to no novel visual stimulation, just field after field of corn and soy. I logically understood the importance of agriculture, having spent some of my childhood on my grandparents' hog farm, but I just couldn't make myself appreciate it in this context.

The flowers always stood out to me. Occasionally interspersed among the grass, often in the ditches, were beautiful patches of pinkish-purple intermixed with white. They were among the only spots of color in a sea of mostly greens and browns. The patches were always small, no more than a few feet wide. Every year when we made the trip, as soon as I grew tired of my books and my games and inevitably resorted to just staring out the window aimlessly, I'd look for the flowers. They were always one of the highlights of an otherwise drab, understimulating landscape.

It was out of character for me, but on one of our drives something compelled me to share my feelings about the flowers.

"Dad, what are those? They're so pretty."

"Some kind of invasive species. They aren't supposed to be there."

I had no idea what an invasive species was, but the term became embedded in my conscious for reasons I didn't understand at the time. It refers to organisms that belong in one ecosystem but are introduced to another, whether accidentally or intentionally. Each region of the world has a unique configuration of plants and animals that sustainably interact with one another to produce a balanced, harmonious environment. When something from another ecosystem is introduced, it throws off the balance of the system and causes problems. Sometimes the effects are devastating.

These flowers weren't originally part of the North American Midwestern ecosystem. They were imported from Asia and Africa, primarily for erosion control. Nature being the wild, uncontrollable force that it is, their seeds dispersed in the wind. Now the flowers were spreading across the highway in intermittent patches, growing well outside of the contained spaces where they were originally planted.

I didn't see what the problem was. So what if they weren't here originally? They were pleasant to look at, especially planted among such a boring, brown backdrop. They made the area more beautiful, more vibrant, and more interesting. They seemed to me like a much-needed source of novelty, and I considered the drive slightly more tolerable because of them.

They didn't have thorns. They weren't poisonous. (I later learned that this is not entirely true; the flower called "crown vetch" actually is poisonous to horses, and only horses, in "large quantities." So please don't allow your horse to binge eat beautiful ditch flowers or it may become terribly ill.) There was absolutely nothing overtly bad, problematic, or dangerous about them.

But not all invasive species cause problems through directly damaging other living organisms. Many, like the crown vetch, are mostly harmless on a small scale. The issue is that they almost never remain small in scale. They cause problems simply by growing unchecked, increasing in number and scope until they become the most prevalent, most dominant species in a region.

At first I thought that sounded wonderful! Imagine an entire field of beautiful flowers. What could be better than that? It wasn't like somebody brought lions to Iowa. It was just a flower.

I didn't grasp the scope of problems an invasive species like crown vetch can create. They cause indirect harm by competing with native grasses. Every ecosystem has a vast, but ultimately finite, supply of resources. Every patch of soil and every ounce of rain is distributed among the inhabitants of the ecosystem. Anything that doesn't belong there takes resources away from something that does. Every inch of space taken up by these flowers was an inch not taken up by a native grass or plant.

While the loss of a single patch of grass wasn't going to destroy an entire ecosystem, it was still causing harm. Most animals won't consume non-native plants, so they provide no value to an environment they've been artificially introduced to beyond looking pretty. They don't functionally interact with the other organisms in the ecosystem and form a dead zone where nothing of value is produced. Too many of these ecological dead zones can throw an entire region into a downward spiral and wipe out entire species due to a lack of resources, as the most fundamental building blocks of the food chain are suddenly in short supply.

A slight reduction in prairie grass means a slight reduction in food for the grasshoppers, which in turn means a slight reduction in the population of grasshoppers. Fewer grasshoppers mean fewer mice. Fewer mice mean fewer foxes, bobcats, and owls. That's how a small, beautiful patch of flowers can kill an apex predator.

And it can also kill a horse if the horse eats too much of it. I'm still not over that.

In other words, the flowers cause harm by taking resources from the environment and giving nothing back. They aren't directly damaging to anything; their biggest crime is being useless while taking up space that could otherwise be occupied by something useful. Too many useless things in an ecosystem tends to destroy the useful things in it.

This lesson was repeated for me later in life with zebra mussels. As their name suggests, they are dark-gray-and-white striped freshwater mollusks. Like the crown vetch, zebra mussels are an invasive species that didn't originally exist in North America. Other than sometimes having sharp edges on their shells, which can hurt if you step on them, they don't cause any direct, obvious harm. They also filter algae from the water, increasing the clarity and visibility of the bodies of water they're found in.

Again, I struggled to understand the problem here. While my parents openly dreaded the day the mussels inevitably found their way to our lake, as they had to many others nearby, tracked in by some careless or clueless boater, I secretly hoped for it. I loved looking into the water and visually locating fish, turtles, frogs, and anything else of interest. Clearer water sounded amazing!

And yet again, I had failed to understand the problem. While not appealing to look at, algae was a critical part of the lake's food chain. It was consumed by water insects and minnows, which were then eaten by larger fish like bass and pike. Less algae meant fewer bugs and minnows, which meant fewer larger fish. A lake overpopulated with zebra mussels would be a big, beautiful, empty lake full of nothing. Basically, a giant swimming pool full of moderately sharp shells.

Outward beauty and visual intrigue are not the indicators of a healthy, thriving ecosystem. An environment that is built to last is an environment with a lot of redundancy and repetition. The most critical, fundamental components of an ecosystem that keep it sustainable are rarely the most interesting or exciting. In fact, it's almost always the opposite.

It is the mundane, the routine, and the familiar that supports life and provides balance. It's the grass in a prairie. It's the ants in a forest. It's the farmland in the heartland. It's everything we overlook and take for granted every single day.

The balance between organisms in an ecosystem is intricate and delicate. It can be thrown off, or even destroyed, by the presence of something that was never intended to be there, even if the greatest crime committed by the invasive species is to simply exist in a place it was never meant to be.

The Lesson

Invasive Species

Like a lake full of zebra mussels, it's all too easy for us to end up with big, beautiful lives full of absolutely nothing. We so often trade the fundamental for the entertaining, the integral for the exciting, and our natural inner balance and harmony collapse as a result.

Our personal ecosystems are even more intricate and even more delicate than the fragile external environments we inhabit. Our thoughts, feelings, and behaviors interact to form a harmonious, sustainable system. Or at least, that's what they're supposed to do.

After a decade of deep depression, I had a few very good years in my early twenties. Finding joy in life and making real progress towards my goals during a time I didn't even expect to be alive was exhilarating. Every moment felt like a blessing, and every day I was pleasantly surprised to find that I wanted to do it all over again tomorrow. Unfortunately, these feelings did not last forever. Life has this annoying habit of changing the rules to the game every time you start to understand them.

The novelty of miraculously becoming a semifunctional adult was beginning to wear off. Like the middle of a long trip, the reality of what I'd committed to was beginning to sink in. Part of why I wasn't sure I ever wanted to participate in adult life was because so much of it seemed like a thankless grind, and unfortunately it was very much starting to feel that way. No major milestones or benchmarks were anywhere in sight. All I saw when I looked forward was months, if not years, of repetitive yet challenging days. It reminded me of our childhood road trips when I was fully aware that there were hundreds of miles of unremarkable terrain between us and our eventual destination.

I started to notice a series of changes inside of me, the symptoms of an illness I had yet to diagnose. Joy became a very acute experience. There were moments of joy to be sure, but existence in and of itself did not feel particularly enjoyable. It wasn't actively unpleasant or torturous as it was in my younger days. This time it felt like nothing at all. I wasn't miserable; I just wasn't *anything*. I felt no particular reaction, positive or negative, to my continued existence.

My goal for each day was simply to endure. As soon as my eyes would open in the morning, I'd be looking forward to the end of the day and the few little distractions I'd find along the way. The escapes, the activities that distracted me from how unenjoyable it was to be me, were the only parts of the day that made me feel anything.

It became difficult to tell my days apart. Other than the broad distinctions between weekdays and weekends, I often couldn't tell you if it was Tuesday or Thursday. They all felt the same to me. My life seemed to happen in much longer blocks of time: weeks, months, or even years. I'd constantly lose track of time during the day. If I had a deadline for a task or a paper, two or three hours would have gone by whenever I checked the clock, and precious minutes seemed to be lost every time I'd blink. On the days when I wasn't working on anything particularly important, the mornings would last approximately twenty hours, and the afternoons felt like about thirty more.

Life felt chronically shallow, like I wasn't really able to connect with anything. I had a young career, an adequate home, and a growing family but didn't feel any real sense of happiness or achievement. Each day was nothing more than a series of disconnected tasks on a to-do list. Wake up. Get ready for work. Work. Eat. Work more. Come home. Cook. Eat. Try to keep everyone around me happy, often unsuccessfully. Go to bed. Do it again the next day. I used to think I'd never be able to do any of these things, but now that I realized I could, I wasn't sure if I cared to.

I was constantly on edge. If everything in my day went exactly the way I hoped and planned for, I was probably OK. Probably. But if anything was harder or took longer than I expected, both of which happened often, I'd fall apart. Sometimes "falling apart" meant picking a stupid fight about nothing. Sometimes it meant pulling away out of shame and frustration. Sometimes it meant not being able to sleep until two in the morning because I couldn't stop thinking about every mistake I'd ever made and how a person with a past like mine shouldn't have anyone or anything depending on them.

Although I didn't gain a significant amount of weight during this time, my body felt distinctly heavier. I was oddly aware of the Earth's gravity and I couldn't shake the feeling that someone had somehow increased it by about 50 percent. Anything that involved moving my body or expending physical energy became incredibly unappealing. I felt almost magnetically pulled down into couches and chairs.

It always felt like I was at least a little bit sick even when I didn't seem to have any diagnosable illness. I hadn't felt "good" or fully healthy in a long time. Aches, pains, and stiffness just seemed like a normal part of life that I attributed to age. I always seemed to be just a little bit short of breath.

My instinctual response to anything I didn't absolutely have to do was a "no." I'd always try to find ways to get out of as many obligations and responsibilities as possible. There was absolutely no room in my emotional budget for any additional expenses. I wasn't even sure if I could afford what I'd already committed to. Every day was taking a little bit more out of me than I could put back in.

The worse these mystery symptoms became, the more I increased my treatment. I could only assume that I was experiencing burnout, or at least a precursor to it, so I took more frequent and longer breaks. I tried to adjust my work-to-leisure ratio to skew a little more favorably towards leisure. Sometimes my days were so packed that my only opportunities for "me time" were late into the night, occasionally even stretching into the early morning.

When this still didn't correct the imbalance, I began cutting things out of my life. I stopped going to the gym, no longer feeling like I had the time or energy for it. I did much less cooking, relying more on fast food and frozen meals. Any efforts to maintain relationships outside of my immediate family were abandoned. I did everything I could think of to strip my life down to what I thought were the bare essentials: providing for my family and de-stressing from providing for my family.

The more I increased my treatment, the worse my symptoms became. When I finally figured it out, I felt like an idiot. The answer had been blatantly obvious for years.

The treatment was the disease.

I wasn't suffering because I was busy or because my life had challenges. Both of those things were certainly true, but everybody's life is like that. I was suffering because I had convinced myself that I needed multiple hours per day of downtime to cope with the inherent stressors of my life. Trying to jam these activities into a life that was already filled to capacity resulted in things being squeezed out. Things that I legitimately needed to stay healthy and functional. Things like sleep, quality nutrition, relationships, and physical activity, the native species in my ecosystem.

Anytime my life has become particularly difficult, my go-to coping tool has always been video games. I've had my flings with shopping and substances, but nothing captivates my mind quite like gaming. I'm not passionate about French wines or Cuban cigars, but a good Japanese role-playing game lights up the pleasure center of my brain like nothing else in this world does. Video games capture my full attention, and for the time I'm engaged with them my problems melt away.

And that's exactly why gaming, at least for me, was the problem.

I logically understand that my friends, my family, my career, and my health are more important than video games. But the reward center of the brain does not distribute dopamine based on morality or importance. Dopamine is based on stimulation, attention follows dopamine, and nothing is more stimulating to my mind than video games.

Left to my own devices, I've found myself in ruts when playing video games eight, ten, even twelve hours a day was common. I've missed hours of sleep to play video games. I've skipped meals to play video games. I've turned down social outings to play video games. I've ignored important chores and tasks to play video games.

Most shamefully, I've ignored my own family to play video games. Growing up, I often rejected invitations to play with my siblings or interact with my parents. In the early years of my marriage, many beautiful weekends were sadly spent indoors staring at a screen rather than enjoying the beautiful forests, lakes, rivers, and small towns of Minnesota with my equally beautiful wife.

But the moment when I couldn't hide behind my denial any longer came the day after my daughter was born. She was our second child, and I learned from the birth of our first that there's a lot more downtime than you expect when you're in the hospital with a newborn. I was prepared this time and brought a handheld gaming system with me, essentially approaching this unique moment of my life in much the same way I approached the long road trips of my childhood: as something to be endured rather than appreciated.

On the night of her birth, everything went well. Although nine days early, she arrived quickly (it seemed that way to me anyway—my wife might disagree) and with a shocking amount of hair. We went to sleep that night as elated parents. Midway through her first full day of life on the outside, we discovered she had a significant birth defect. We were transferred to the NICU and told she would likely need to be taken to a larger hospital for a surgical procedure. Our lives had turned completely upside down in an hour.

Before we left to follow the ambulance in our own car (we weren't allowed to ride with her for reasons I still don't understand), I threw my handheld gaming console in the garbage. In that moment, I could no longer justify the cost. We weren't sure if she was going to make it (note: she did and is generally doing well today), and the realization that I had spent some of what might have been her very limited time on Earth distracted by silly games made me physically ill. I couldn't stop thinking of everything I'd sacrificed in life for one more hour of digital stimulation. That was the day I vowed to begin weeding out my own invasive species.

If you had known me before then, I wouldn't have told you that gaming was a problem for me. Quite the opposite. I'd have clung firmly to my assertion that gaming was the only thing keeping me going. On the particularly hard days, my solo time with my PC was the only part I looked forward to. That's exactly how it was ruining my life.

What happened over the next few years defied every expectation I had. There was, as expected, a withdrawal period when I had no idea what to do with myself. When my to-do list was empty and nobody needed me, I utterly lacked direction and mostly just wandered around the house aimlessly, randomly moving objects from one place to another. These occasional pockets of free time perplexed me, as they would normally have gone to gaming.

For a few weeks I felt about as low as I could recall in recent years. My life had just as many tasks and responsibilities as before, but no big reward was waiting for me at the end of the day. It felt like even more of a thankless grind than it already did. This period was extremely challenging, and I will not sugarcoat that. My brain was rewiring itself to find pleasure in other things, and the gap in which it hadn't found anything was emotionally excruciating. Thankfully, this didn't last very long. As the turmoil wore off and I acclimated to my new way of living, I noticed the reemergence of an emotion I hadn't felt in years: boredom! For the first time in well over a decade, I had more time and energy than my days required of me, and I didn't know how to spend the surplus.

I decided to try reinvesting my suddenly abundant time and energy into everything I had abandoned rather than trying to immediately find a new, less addictive hobby. I worked on reestablishing a good sleep routine, a healthy relationship with food, and regular daily physical activity. I spent more time with my family and didn't rush through whatever they wanted to do because I wanted to get to what I wanted to do. I also began taking on "side hustles" like social media and writing books. For the first time, I truly had nothing better to do than take care of my health, be with my family, and work on advancing my career.

It wasn't shocking to me that these changes made me healthier, but it was extremely shocking to me that they also made me happier. I found myself able to enjoy most of my days for the first time since I was a child, days which once again felt distinct from one another. My sense of connection to my family and my work became much stronger. The irritability and tension began to fade. I felt lighter, more energized, and more comfortable in my body. Life no longer felt like a grind I was just enduring my way through. Although I was thrilled by this outcome, I struggled to understand how, exactly, I had achieved it. How could removing the part of my life that I enjoyed most make me enjoy my life more rather than less?

After taking some time to reflect on this period, I developed a theory that I try to live by to this day: If there's anything in my life that feels dramatically "better" than everything else I have to do, it will ultimately make me less happy to include that activity in my life than to live without it. Anytime I'm not doing that thing, I will wish I was doing that thing and therefore find it difficult, if not impossible, to enjoy whatever I am currently doing.

This, I believe, is the basis of all behavioral addictions. Our brains want to do the thing that feels best as often as possible. and they get at least a little upset, and sometimes a lot upset, when they haven't been able to do that thing for a while. We end up craving those experiences and resenting everything that gets in the way of them, even if what "gets in the way" is something objectively more important such as people we love, things we need to do to stay healthy, or religious practices that provide us with a sense of purpose.

And that's how my life improved dramatically when I removed my favorite part of it. This subtraction paradoxically became a massive addition because it elevated my enjoyment of every other part of my life, which ultimately took up much more of my time than gaming was ever going to. Improving my enjoyment of everything moved the needle significantly more than constantly chasing one optimally enjoyable thing. I pulled the weeds, gained more resources by doing so, and redistributed those resources to more fundamental parts of my life.

If I thought this was some unique brain glitch that only worked on me (which is a possibility I always consider), I wouldn't be writing a chapter about it. I'm confident in what I'm saying here because I've seen this pattern play out over and over again in the lives of other people.

If you studied my therapy clients who have made and maintained the most progress, you would observe a set of solid fundamentals at their foundation. Some of them are the practices we covered in the first chapter of this book: They prioritize getting an adequate amount of sleep whenever possible at as close to the same time every night as possible. They nourish their bodies and minds with high-quality caloric energy on a predictable schedule. They engage in regular physical activity to keep blood and oxygen pumping as efficiently as possible throughout the body and the brain. Then, they also minimize or avoid any substances that create peaks and valleys in their mood or their energy level. They value stability and consistency over acute moments of joy or excitement.

Not only do they do these things consistently and well, but they enjoy doing these things. Taking excellent care of themselves is a hobby. Feeling better physically and mentally is their primary goal in life, taking precedence over activities with no purpose beyond producing a single, acute moment of pleasant emotions. They have little desire to closely follow the lives of others on television or social media because all their needs are met through simply living their own lives and taking excellent care of themselves.

Put another way, hobbies work best when they're used to fill in the cracks between the important parts of our lives, an outlet for energy when nothing important is happening. When our hobbies become so important to us that life itself starts to feel like the cracks we have to fill, things have gone too far.

Ultimately, this isn't a lesson about video game addiction. This is a lesson about how the things we love most tend to take over and potentially ruin our lives, just like too many beautiful flowers on a prairie can ruin that ecosystem. My flowers just happen to be video games.

So we've talked about mine. Now let's talk about yours.

The Application

Managing Your Ecosystem

We're all just trying to find ways to cope with the drudgery of the middle of our respective journeys. The period of life after the shine and sparkle of childhood has faded, but the next major milestone seems impossibly far off on the horizon. There are moments of immense joy and excitement in the middle, but we're all searching for ways to fill the gaps in between. What we plant in these empty spaces can destroy our lives.

Sometimes we allow invasive species to take root in these gaps. We, too, have non-native inhabitants that compete for our resources. Vibrant, exciting bursts of stimulation that provide no substantial long-term value to our lives. Like beautiful flowers in a ditch, these things are functionally harmless in small quantities but tend to burst free from their boundaries to take over and dominate our lives.

Our native species are the things we must do, the nonnegotiable parts of life. Going to work or school. Maintaining our bodies and our environments. Spending time with our families. Spiritual practices. The core elements of life that keep you healthy, functional, and energized. They put resources back into our environment, like leaves converting carbon dioxide into breathable air, and keep our inner ecosystems running sustainably.

Like the endless identical blades of grass in a prairie or the thousands of indistinguishable ants in a colony, these inescapable parts of our lives aren't particularly novel or glamorous. Even if they once were, they quickly lose their stimulation value when the novelty wears off. Because these parts of life are routine, sometimes even mundane, it's easy for them to feel unimportant. They don't have the excitement or the novelty of a patch of beautiful, colorful flowers in an otherwise bland-looking prairie.

Invasive species are the behaviors that don't provide any essential functions to our ecosystem. All they do is fill the space where other things should be. They produce nothing in your life beyond momentary pleasure. They create a single temporary pocket of joy, then quickly disappear into nonexistence. At best, they have no long-term impact on your life. At worst, they begin to destroy it.

These behaviors create functional dead zones in your day where nothing of value is produced. Centering your life on these behaviors puts you in a never-ending cycle of pursuit, a constant loop of craving the next source of the excitement that distracts you from the turmoil or the emptiness inside. When invasive species begin to outcompete native species, the delicate balance that is our lives begins to fall apart.

The difference between the experience of a person who has effectively cultivated the native inhabitants of their inner ecosystem and a person who has allowed invasive species to run rampant can be summarized as this: The former feels as good as they're capable of feeling at each and every moment of the day because their resources are optimized, while the latter is in constant pursuit of the next experience that feels "good" and endures, if not dreads, the spaces in between. If you're the latter type of person, this chapter is for you.

There's nothing inherently wrong with doing something just because it feels good, but these behaviors so easily grow to uncontrollable proportions and can so easily take over our lives entirely. They're usually introduced in a contained manner: a midday break to prevent burnout or an evening reward for a hard day's work. But, like the seeds of an invasive flower blowing across a prairie in a windstorm, these hobbies tend to slowly but relentlessly creep into other areas of our lives and steal resources from what truly belongs there.

Sometimes they cause harm that is direct and easily observable. If you're struggling to regulate gambling and shopping, you can visibly tally the damage every time you check your bank account. A problem with food, substances, or self-harm takes a toll on a person that is often visible to others. But more often than not, the damage they cause is beneath the surface.

There is nothing morally wrong with watching football, for example. You work hard and you absolutely deserve, and need, to rest. Watching sports is not a problematic or inappropriate way to accomplish this. However, if your need to rest via sports grows into a deep fandom and a compulsive desire to watch every single game and study the teams extensively between watching games, the quality of your life is inevitably going to decline. There simply aren't enough resources in your life, time, and energy to nurture such a demanding hobby while maintaining everything you need to thrive, and something more fundamental to your overall well-being is going to get squeezed out as a consequence.

Playing video games every day will not directly harm your body, nor will it inherently make you more depressed or anxious (other than acutely, such as when you lose a game of *Madden* to a trash-talking nine-year-old. Please don't ask me how I know this). But playing video games for hours a day will indirectly result in a decline in your physical and mental health and a corresponding net decrease in your quality of life that outweighs the increase in quality of life that comes from the gaming itself. You'll inevitably start to prioritize gaming over meeting your needs and taking care of your responsibilities because gaming is so much more immediately enjoyable and stimulating.

Your ecosystem may be resilient to electronic stimulation such as gaming or social media, but I'm certain it has at least one major vulnerability. You probably already know what it is. For some of us it's a substance like marijuana, alcohol, or something harder. For others it's food, whether consuming it, avoiding it, or getting rid of it after consuming it. For many people it's money, whether spending it, working endlessly to hoard it, or gambling it away.

All of these behaviors are self-perpetuating. The more time you spend on them, the further you drift from the person you want to be and the life you wish you had. This gap between ideal and real creates emotional distress that demands soothing. You soothe it by using the most rewarding behavior. And that's how you eventually find yourself scrolling social media on the toilet for thirty minutes while avoiding your actual life and wishing you were someone else.

There's only one way out of this cycle, and it's probably going to sound like a terrible idea unless you understand how your enjoyment of the things you do in your life is a dynamic variable rather than a static variable. Dynamic variables change depending on what else is happening around them, but static variables never change and are unaffected by whatever happens around them. Your enjoyment of the things you do is a dynamic variable.

The weather is a perfect example of this. If it's fifty-five degrees outside today, that is a static variable. The temperature is simply the temperature, and it doesn't really care what you think or feel about it. How you experience that temperature is a dynamic variable.

A fifty-five-degree day in the Midwestern United States in January feels almost tropical, a welcome reprieve from the single-digit or subzero temperatures that are common in this region at that time of year. People will celebrate in the streets in shorts and T-shirts. Grills will be ignited. Mother Nature will be praised. We will all feel blessed. The meteorologist will call it a top-ten weather day.

A fifty-five-degree day in the same region in early April feels "average." It's what is expected and feels neither particularly warm nor particularly cool. It's simply a normal weather day and usually doesn't evoke strong feelings from anyone.

A fifty-five-degree day in the same region in mid-July feels frigid. These days make you question what, exactly, God might be punishing you for. People will stay inside at all costs. When forced to go outside they will bundle up in winter clothing as if they're in danger of frostbite.

The variation in our physical, mental, and emotional reactions to a situation that is objectively the same across all three situations is primarily a product of comparison. The same temperature feels dramatically warmer in winter and dramatically colder in summer because of how it compares to the days before and after it.

Everything in our lives works like this. Whether something feels "good," "bad," or just "normal" is almost entirely based on what we compare it to, and what we compare it to is almost always the best and worst parts of our current lives.

For me, gaming is a ten out of ten on the enjoyment scale. It creates the "good" comparison point in my life when it's a part of my life. The reason that gaming is so destructive to my internal ecosystem is that it pushes all of the things I have to do to around a five on the same scale. That's how much my brain loves gaming.

Time with friends and family is about a six. Working out and cooking are around a five. Work itself is typically a four, as are cleaning and housework. Everything I do pales in comparison. Because I have to do most of these things every day, my average enjoyment of any given moment hovers at around a "five" with the occasional "ten" thrown in, usually at the end of the day.

Without gaming, my anchor points reset. Something must always be a ten, and after a period of de-habituation from an exceptionally stimulating activity, the next best thing becomes your ten. In my case, it's time with friends and family. Because everything else I have to do is only a point or two below friends and family on the enjoyment scale, everything else moves up, because it's now being compared to time with friends and family instead of gaming and, sadly, the gap isn't nearly as wide. Working out and cooking are now a nine. Cleaning and housework become an eight. My enjoyment of an average day increases massively as a result.

Acting like an addict is no longer the exclusive territory of people who use hard drugs regularly. The optional parts of life, the invasive species introduced to our lives by profit-driven corporations, have become so stimulating that our native species, the things we must do to survive and thrive, cannot compete and are being overtaken. I firmly believe that nearly every human being alive is addicted to something, and it's almost impossible not to be at this point.

My definition of addiction is admittedly a bit broader than most. For me, an addiction is anything that I prioritize over the most important parts of my life. In other words, if I regularly choose something over going to bed when I'm tired, eating when I'm hungry, being with my loved ones when I have the opportunity, and generally taking optimal care of my body, mind, and soul, I consider myself addicted to that thing and work to minimize or eliminate its presence in my life.

This may sound extreme, but please consider it in the context of the direction our society seems to be heading in. How often do you hear people lament that there simply aren't enough hours in the day to do what needs to be done? These complaints often come from people with daily screen time averages of three, four, or even five-plus hours. If you don't have time to do the things you need to do, what other possible solution could there be other than to do less of the things you don't actually need to do?

This is not some unsolvable problem—it's an inevitable experience of the human condition. If the previous paragraph described you, please know that you aren't alone. It is culturally normal to fall into patterns of chronic self-neglect. The average adult in America needs eight hours of sleep each night but gets six and a half. We function best by eating at least three meals per day, yet we average just two. Fewer than half of us meet the recommended physical activity guidelines of 150 minutes of exercise per week, and nearly a third of us report getting no significant physical activity at all on a regular basis. Two-thirds of us regularly consume alcohol for purposes of mood regulation, and more than half of us are dependent upon consuming caffeine at least once per day, and in most cases several times per day, in order to have enough energy to function. Collectively, we are in rough shape.

The average adult in America is also not very happy. In a 2021 survey, the average self-reported life satisfaction score was a 6.89 on a ten-point scale. Converted into a letter grade, that's the equivalent of a D+. Do you want to live a 6.89 type of life? I'm guessing not, or else you probably wouldn't be reading this. If you don't want to live a D+ life, you can't study like the other D+ students. You aren't so different or so special that you can neglect your own needs just like most people neglect their own needs yet somehow achieve a better outcome than they do. If you want a better life, you have to find a better way to live.

Every year, more and more distractions and recreational opportunities become available to us. Social media channels number in the hundreds of millions, and many of them have the production values of a Hollywood movie. Video games become dramatically more immersive and realistic. Every distraction pulling us away from our "mundane" lives becomes more accessible and more appealing. We have an entire universe at our fingertips every second of every day.

In middle school, my class was tasked with writing an essay describing our dream houses. Mine had, among other things, a "gaming library" (because of course it did) that contained every Super Nintendo game ever made. It seemed like an impossible dream at the time. I could have that room on my phone now if I wanted to.

Despite this, we do not appear to be becoming happier. Life satisfaction is such a complicated variable that it's difficult to fully assess, but self-reported measures of subjective quality of life year after year suggest either a stagnation or a gradual decline in global subjective happiness. We are on a happiness plateau at best, a gradual downhill slide at worst.

If we're constantly adding more and more things to our existence that distract us from our problems, yet becoming less and less happy year over year, what does that tell us?

I know what it tells me: that distracting ourselves, no matter how shiny the trinket, is never the solution. In fact, I think it's the problem. The solution is to live our actual lives and take care of our actual bodies and minds. To nurture and attend to the legitimate needs that are native to our well-being, while stemming the rampant growth of invasive habits that so quickly and easily become the centerpieces of our lives.

We try to find ways around it, tricks, "hacks," and strategies to avoid doing the hard, obvious thing. But there isn't a way around it.

Well-known financial advisor Dave Ramsey often says, "If you want to live like nobody else, you have to live like nobody else." I don't know if that's a Dave Ramsey original quote or if he's quoting someone else, but I heard him say it first, so I'm calling it a Dave Ramsey quote. He's talking about money, his point being that you can't spend like everyone else and enjoy a greater degree of financial security than most people have, but this quote applies to everything. If you live like other people, you will feel like other people, and most people don't like their lives very much.

It was extremely obvious to me what was draining all of my time and energy away, but I'm aware that some people's invasive species are far more subtle than mine. I don't want anything to sneak in under your radar, so I'm going to introduce some terms that will help you weed out anything you want gone.

Anything that reduces your emotional distress is a coping tool. Coping tools are neither inherently good nor bad, healthy nor unhealthy. Like any tool, their effectiveness depends mostly on how they are used.

There are two types of coping tools: self-care and self-distraction. I'm going to tell you how I define them, which doesn't necessarily match what you're probably thinking of right now. What much of the world considers to be self-care, I consider to be self-distraction. This distinction is crucial because these two categories of behaviors serve very different roles in our lives, and mixing them up will keep you feeling hopelessly stuck.

Self-care actions are behaviors that fundamentally change what it feels like to inhabit your mind and your body in a permanent or semipermanent matter. In other words, these are behaviors that make you mentally and/or physically healthier. Improving your sleep hygiene is self-care. Practicing gratitude is self-care. Strengthening your relationships is self-care. Being physically active is self-care. Mindfulness is self-care. Meditation is self-care. Spiritual practices are self-care. This is by no means an exhaustive list, just a few from among hundreds of potential examples.

Self-care activities should be your primary focus every day, because they are ultimately the only actions you can take that improve the conditions of your inner ecosystem. They are your only method of restoring or enhancing your access to the world. In general they are more work than self-distraction activities and create less of an immediate sense of reward, but they build up over time because they pay off more than once. More on this later.

Self-distractions are behaviors that make you temporarily less aware of how unpleasant it currently feels to be you. They don't change how it feels to be you; they simply take your attention away from your current reality for a time. Drugs and alcohol are self-distractions. Video games and television are self-distractions. Social media is, for the most part, a self-distraction. Again, not an exhaustive list, just a few examples.

It isn't bad, wrong, or unhelpful to self-distract. Sometimes you need it. It's unrealistic to expect a person to do nothing but practice self-improvement every day. Life can be overwhelming, and sometimes we just need to disconnect for a while. There's no shame in that. None.

But for so many people, these distractions become the primary focal point of their lives. If they are your only coping mechanism, your mind is gradually falling into a state of disrepair because self-distraction alone doesn't fundamentally change what's inside of you. In fact, you might notice that you need an ever-increasing frequency or intensity of distractions to produce the relief you're hoping for. This is because your inner distress is growing, and you're doing nothing to stop or reduce the growth. What you're trying to distract yourself from is getting bigger and bigger, so the distractions need to become bigger and bigger in proportion to the distress.

There's no way to permanently escape the experience of being yourself while you're still alive. Our world is filled with things that promise a temporary escape from stress and pain, but that's all they're ever capable of being. You can distract yourself from what it feels like to live inside of yourself, but you can never depart from your mind and your body. And, so often, it is the act of distracting from the experience of existing within yourself that prevents you from improving the experience of existing within yourself. The distractions from the unpleasantness also serve as distractions from the solution.

Please note that that is *not* me casting judgment on you or telling you that you need to be a "productive member of society." As you have probably gathered by now, I am not exactly a member of the human society fan club. I don't feel a tremendously strong urge to give back to society considering that the main thing society has given me could be summarized as "complexes." I'm simply informing you how your brain works.

I'm also not suggesting that you should remove every optional source of joy from your life and become some sort of monk with a job. Actually, maybe being a monk is considered a job, in which case that sentence was incredibly invalidating to monks. Either way, the scale of your life is immense, and trying to micromanage every little detail of it would be like trying to weed a thousand-acre forest—an exercise in frustration and futility. You don't need to examine your life with a microscope. I just want you to consider pulling the weeds that are taking up huge chunks of your mental ecosystem and giving you nothing in return.

There's a war going on inside of you every day, and you cannot win that war by trying to escape it. You can never escape what is inside of you. In addition, the act of retreating inward takes you further away from the world and even deeper into yourself. If you're stuck in patterns of psychological self-abuse and invalidation, retreating deeper into your mind is moving in the wrong direction.

If your life has been taken over by something that isn't native to your ecosystem, we need to take drastic action to remove it. The problem will not resolve on its own. When I let invasive species into my ecosystem, they inevitably outcompete my genuine needs. They are simply too stimulating and too engaging to stay contained within a harmless little corner of my life. The only way I've been able to maintain a quality of life that I find acceptable to is do my best to avoid exposure to them and to weed them out whenever I find them.

My fourth lesson to you is this: Pull the weeds that are stealing the water and sunlight from the most important parts of your life. The thing you love doing the most might actually be the very thing that is ruining your life. If so, I want you to consider eliminating it from your ecosystem entirely and treating it like the invasive species that it is.

Truth Five

Love What You Have

The Story

The Farm

Only once in my life have I cried so hard I thought I might die. Driving alone at night on an empty Nebraska highway, the ugly sobs felt like they could rip my heart out of my chest. I should have pulled over, should have taken as much time as I needed to let it all out rather than continuing to drive with eyes so drenched they needed their own set of windshield wipers. I just wanted to get to the hotel as quickly as possible so that I could fully collapse into my emotions without having to multitask. George Strait's "Blue Clear Sky" coming from the speakers taunted me with the promise of happiness I thought I might never experience again.

I had just come from the farm. Or, rather, what used to be the farm. It hadn't looked the way I remembered it.

Every day on the farm was a good day until the day it wasn't anymore.

Each farm morning began with a distinct aroma. No, not that one. It was the unmistakable smell of bacon frying in the pan, which my grandmother dutifully prepared as soon as the sun rose. The little farmhouse couldn't have been more than a thousand square feet, and every inch of it filled up with that wonderful, smoky/sweet aroma every morning. It reached all three bedrooms, the family room, the living room, the lone bathroom, and of course the kitchen itself.

The sharp metallic "clang" of the lids on the hog feeders and the sound of the bacon sizzling combined to create the morning soundtrack. Surrounding the farmhouse on two sides were dozens of hog pens. The feeders were large, metallic cylinders with lids that the hogs could lift up with their snouts, allowing them to feed on demand throughout the day. Hogs rise with the sun and, like some of us, wake up hungry. They are not dainty creatures, so anytime one finished eating, the lid that was previously resting on its head would come crashing down. The loud metal-on-metal sound could be jarring if you weren't used to it. To me, it was a soothing reminder that the long car ride from eastern Iowa to southern Nebraska really happened, and my memory of arriving at the farm in the middle of the dark night wasn't a dream. We were really back.

No work was to be done on an empty stomach. Breakfast was always bacon and cereal for me and my siblings, a mix of whatever store-brand offering my grandmother happened to buy to prepare for our arrival and, for some reason, Grape-Nuts. Always Grape-Nuts. They invariably sank to the bottom of the bowl, but if you were patient enough, they'd absorb some sugary goodness from the children's cereal hovering in the milk above them. My personal favorite was Cinni-Mini-Crunch, which, if the marketing team had been honest, would have been called "Cinnamon Toast Crunch if you left the box open for a day." Our grandfather always had the stereotypical full farmer's breakfast with bacon, eggs, and buttered toast. He also salted his toast—probably not the healthiest practice, but one I've stolen from him and retain to this day.

Next came chores. We'd grab our "feed buckets" (repurposed five-gallon plastic ice-cream containers) and take them out to the silo and fill them with hog feed. Systematically, we went to every hog pen and gave the animals their breakfasts. Some were fed in the aforementioned metal feeders with lids, some in troughs, and some simply in a line on the ground. The hogs always grunted their appreciation while they ate. Hearing their joy made me feel like there was a purpose to our toiling.

Our grandfather always gave us cardinal directions to the pens, which I was never able to memorize. When I was younger, I would just walk off in some random direction to see if he corrected me or not, but eventually I discovered that there was a metal rooster-topped weathervane above the barn that I could use as a reference point. The chores took a while, but they needed to be completed no matter how we felt. We fed the hogs in the rain, the snow, and the sweltering heat.

Our reward for completion was always the same: a cold Mountain Dew and a Hershey's bar, with or without almonds (I always chose "with") straight out of the fridge in the barn. I'm not exactly sure why they kept the Hershey's bars in the fridge, but every year on the anniversary of my grandmother's death I buy a six-pack of almond Hershey's and a bottle of Mountain Dew and throw them in the fridge to be savored. When the first bite of cold chocolate hits my mouth, I'm nine years old and carefree once more, if only for an instant. That instant is worth the price of admission every time.

After finishing our chores, we'd usually spend a couple of hours watching television or playing Atari 2600. There was no cable that far from town, so the television signal came in through a massive satellite dish in the front yard that looked like it could probably be used to intercept extraterrestrial communications. We'd binge watch Looney Tunes while enjoying our morning snack, a reward for hard work done well.

There were always more chores in the afternoon. Moving hogs, building fences, pulling weeds, checking on piglets, building or repairing things; the work on a farm is never truly "done," just "done enough for now." Sometimes our grandfather would put the three of us in the scoop bucket on the front of the tractor, raise it to maximum height, and drive us around the farm giving us a bird's-eye view of everything. Not sure how my parents rubber-stamped that one, but miraculously nobody was ever injured.

I could wax poetic for dozens of pages about the beauty and the joy we had on the farm. Driving south to Kansas to pick up fireworks and lighting them in an open field on a warm and humid July night. Keeping a dozen tiny kittens warm in my lap during a blizzard. Leaping across the gaps between seemingly endless rows of hay bales pretending we were all collectively Indiana Jones. Catching dozens of identical yellow bullheads using slices of summer sausage as bait in the little pond just over the hill. Playing hearts and spades on the living room floor in front of the console television. Going into town for burgers, fries, and chicken tenders at the only restaurant for ten miles. I can't even remember everything we did there. The days were always packed.

The farmhouse itself was a warm, happy place full of love and memories. It always seemed brimming with treasure, relics of the past that offered me a little glimpse into what life was like before I entered it. In retrospect my grandparents were at least low-level hoarders and most of what they kept could probably be correctly classified as "junk," but in the eyes of a child it all seemed valuable. Tiny as it was, I loved to explore the farmhouse just to learn more about my grandparents and my dad's childhood.

The lone exception to the cluttered state of their home was my aunt's bedroom. It was tidy and meticulous, perhaps in reaction or defiance to the state of the rest of the house, and it ominously foreshadowed her eventually losing her battle with obsessive-compulsive disorder and anorexia. It looked like it had been grafted on from another house. Something about that specific room always fascinated me. Maybe it was because, like me, it always seemed just a little out of place.

The farm fell just short of northern Minnesota in my "favorite places" hierarchy. I loved everything about it except the smell, and in a fairly extreme example of classical conditioning, the aroma of a hog farm makes me a little misty-eyed because of the memories I associate with it. There are a few hog farms within a five-mile radius of our current home, and when the wind is blowing just right, I can detect the faintest hint of that familiar farm smell in my backyard. In those moments, I feel the nurturing presence of my grandparents once again.

My love for the farm and for my grandparents was immense, but even that love wasn't strong enough to stand against the raging tide of mental illness that began to take over my mind at age thirteen. I brought my Super Nintendo with me for my first trip to the farm as an adolescent, and I spent most of my precious few days there ignoring the usual routines and activities to play video games. The feelings of love, warmth, connection, and excitement that I'd always felt when visiting the farm weren't there for me the way they had been. I interpreted this as a natural sign of growth and maturity, indicators of my inevitable aging out of family-oriented activities.

I was so very wrong about this. I hadn't stopped loving the farm or my grandparents. I wasn't too old to be able to enjoy family time. I was severely depressed and unable to feel much of anything beyond the very acute pleasure from activities like gaming that occasionally broke through the fog of my disorder. What was happening to me was anything but natural. My feelings hadn't changed or disappeared; I just couldn't access them. I realized all of this far too late.

The next three times I visited southern Nebraska were all for funerals. My aunt's, my grandmother's, and then my grandfather's.

The loss of my grandmother hit me the hardest. That's what triggered the aforementioned "crying so hard I thought I might die" spell. Seeing her in her casket during the visitation was the moment I truly realized that it was all over. Not just her life, which was sad enough in and of itself, but everything I wrote about in this chapter. The farm was gone. She was gone. My childhood was gone. And we would never all be together in that place again like we used to be. A decade of deferred grief was condensed into a single moment, as all the feelings I'd been trying so hard to flee from hit me all at once.

I held it together in front of my family somehow, but I broke down in front of George Strait. On that lonely, dark Nebraska highway, I felt every ounce of my pain.

The part that hurt the most was the guilt. It was knowing I could have had nearly another decade of the magic and the wonder of the farm with my family, and I threw it all away for nothing. Teenage me didn't know what was wrong with him or what to do about it. He just knew that nothing in his life made him happy anymore, so he concluded that he needed a new life. He got rid of everything that came before and started over. And now, as an adult, I had to face the consequences of that irreversible decision.

The Lesson

Lost Forever

The loss of my grandmother caused me to spiral into yet another deep depression. This one at least felt a little bit justified. Attending her funeral had finally made tangible the incredible grief of everything my mental illness had taken from me. Although I had achieved a degree of health and stability in adulthood that I never thought possible in my younger years, her death reminded me that there were still holes in my past that could never be filled. Perhaps my relatively few good years had been propped up by unsustainable denial and delusion that were finally rotting and collapsing. What an idiot I was for thinking a person could recover from what I had been through. People like me don't get to have happy endings.

I had lost years, decades in some cases, of potential experiences with the most important people in the world to me during some of the most critical years of my life. Most of my adolescence was spent with "friends" who had long since abandoned me. I had nobody to reminisce with about the relatively few good times I had during those years because everyone who was there for them with me had already left my life. It's amazing how quickly a good memory becomes a tragic one when everyone else who would remember it with you is long gone.

I'd also missed out on making new memories in the parts of this world that were most special to me. I have no stories to tell you about the farm or Minnesota from my adolescence until my early twenties because I wasn't there. I was too busy spending time in dark basements and attics with people who couldn't help me, looking for answers that nobody had to questions I didn't know how to ask.

My withdrawal into the world of isolation and depression had fragmented my family, and those relationships remained strained and damaged two decades later. As the oldest of three siblings, I was a somewhat unwilling role model for my brother and sister. I know they looked up to me immensely, and my rapid and dramatic exit from all family functions set an unfortunate example for them to later follow, which they eventually did in their own ways. That was perhaps what hurt the most; I hadn't just damaged my own life but the lives of others who loved me and relied upon me.

The awareness that I had voluntarily surrendered so many things I could never get back and had absolutely nothing to show for it crushed me. I worried that no matter how hard I worked and how wonderful a life I built in the future, it would never be enough to make up for what I had lost. Every day was haunted by unanswerable questions: What if the best part of my life is already over? What if everything from here on out is nothing more than an endurance race, a test to see how much longer I could keep going before breaking down?

Unfortunately, my grandmother's funeral was only the first of many times life would punch me right in the kidney of regret. It happened again just a few years later, the first time I took my young children to my childhood home in northern Minnesota. I thought this would be a wonderful experience, a chance to relive the best parts of my childhood from the perspective of an adult—and my only opportunity to do so given that the farm was gone.

It was anything but that.

I spent a large chunk of that trip crying. It was my grandmother's funeral all over again, yet another stark reminder of everything my mental illness had taken from me. I couldn't fully enjoy or appreciate the seemingly wonderful experiences my own children were having because I was haunted by ghosts and echoes of what once was—what ended all too early and for the wrong reasons. It felt like a sad, lonely version of my own experiences, the Temu version of my childhood. I couldn't stop thinking about the people who weren't there, those places that were gone, and the many ways it seemed so different from what I saw in my memories. I just wanted to be twelve years old again, fishing and swimming and exploring with my mom, my dad, my brother, and my sister.

Severe irritability and anger often come bundled with depressive episodes, and these were two of the symptoms that hit me the hardest. The worse my mood became, the more annoying I found it to spend time with my loved ones. I couldn't stand to see their faces or hear their voices even when they were doing absolutely nothing wrong. Hearing their footsteps on the hardwood or the sounds of them chewing food or breathing enraged me. It took everything in me not to constantly lash out at them for these perceived slights, and I often failed to keep my anger inside. Somehow, I irrationally blamed them for my misery.

My experiences revisiting Nebraska and Minnesota as an adult taught me that the most normal parts of our lives are often the most important, the ones we will grieve the hardest when they're over. It's difficult to appreciate them when they exist in abundance. We went to Minnesota every year for an entire summer and to the farm for a week at a time once, if not twice, a year. It felt inevitable to my young mind that these would be people and places I could always return to in the future if I needed to. Taking time away from them felt risk free. I always thought I could go back if and when I was ready to do so, like the prodigal son being welcomed back with open arms. By the time I realized I was wrong, most of it was gone.

Grief is painful enough, but the hurt is magnified dramatically when regret and guilt are stacked on top of it. In our naïve, ignorant bliss we tend to subconsciously believe that the best parts of our lives will last forever. We can't face the pain of realizing that every beautiful moment eventually has to end, so we remain steadfast in our denial of the very temporary nature of everything that is precious to us until it's too late.

This causes us to overlook the joy and the wonder that's right in front of our faces. We cannot see what is special, memorable, or noteworthy about our own lives until it is lost. Tragically, that's often the first moment when we finally realize what we've taken for granted.

When certain chapters of our lives close, which is inevitable, we can find ourselves once again experiencing debilitating envy—not for the life of someone else but for the life we once had and took for granted. We desperately long for a fully informed do-over of the best parts of our pasts so that we could appropriately appreciate those unique, irreplaceable moments.

I think this is why antiques and collector's items often end up being absurdly valuable once the people who would have owned them as children are somewhere between thirty and sixty years of age. We're all just chasing the ghosts of our respective childhoods, desperately searching for anything that reminds us of the last time life truly felt good and thinking we can re-create those experiences if we just have the right tools. I have to admit that I would be sorely tempted to pay a completely irrational price for a fresh twelve-pack of Surge and a bag of original Doritos 3D, not because they were culinary delicacies, but because they're intwined in my mind with precious memories I can't fully access.

There's a commonly used therapy technique that involves redirecting maladaptive social comparisons by contrasting your present self with your past self instead of somebody else. I like the concept in general and have used it with many therapy clients with excellent results, but it tends to backfire horribly when I use it on myself. My first instinctual response always seems to be that my past was much, much better than my present.

I spent half a decade of my life chased by ghosts of guilt and regret, ruminating constantly about the people, places, and moments that were lost forever. In an alternate universe, there was a version of myself that continued to visit the farm. He never stopped doing his chores in the morning and eating cold Hershey's bars. He learned more life lessons from the wisest people he knew and modeled those lessons to his little brother and sister. It ruined me that I couldn't give him life, especially knowing that I was the one who killed him.

For a long time, I tried to cope with this pain by attempting to experience what I thought were the closest approximations of the parts of my life that were cut tragically short by mental illness. My hope was to retroactively fill the holes in my heart by creating my own versions of corrective emotional experiences.

I'll give myself some credit for a novel idea with a plausible hypothesis, but it quickly became clear to me that this strategy would never work. Nothing I could create in my present life seemed remotely comparable to the missing parts of the life I left behind. Like the store-brand cereal on the farm, it had the right basic elements, but it was always just a bit "off" in a way that was difficult to articulate. Eventually I gave up on trying, accepting that the damage was permanent and nothing would ever feel the same.

Ironically, this acceptance was the missing piece of my process I didn't know I needed. When I stopped trying to re-create the past, I also stopped comparing the present to the past. It was the comparisons themselves that cheapened my enjoyment of everything good in my adult life. I was creating a second set of missing experiences in my story by longing for the memories of my past while failing to appreciate what was special about the present.

Viewing the past through an emotional lens while looking at my present life through a logical lens created the quality gap that I felt. My perspective alone was the reason everything I had always seemed like a pale imitation of what I'd lost. Nothing could objectively be as good as my memories of the farm felt.

Nothing proves this point more clearly than the farm itself. I know I've made it sound like a very special place, and in my heart it always will be, but objectively it was just a normal farm. So many of my fondest experiences there were objectively unremarkable. Frankly, much of it was dangerous, and some of it was almost certainly in violation of child labor laws. I could have just as easily described it as a hardship of my childhood by focusing on the hard work, the smell, the limited food choices, and the challenges of seven people sharing one bathroom.

It wasn't the farm itself that made these memories so special but the state of mind I was in while at the farm. I wasn't constantly worrying that there was a better farm down the road where I could have had even more fun. Doing what I loved with the people I loved was always enough for me when I was there. That, more than anything, was what I had lost and couldn't seem to reclaim.

But if I had it once, surely I could have it again. I just needed to figure out how.

The Application

Remember What Matters Most

In one of the final episodes of the television show *The Office*, Ed Helms's character, Andy Bernard, makes an oddly profound, serious, and memorable statement about human psychology: "I wish there was a way to know you're in the good old days before you've left them." This quote is often repeated and seems to have struck a nerve with many people. Appreciating what is special before we lose it seems to be a nearly impossible task for the human mind.

I have good news for you. There is a way. In fact, I know several of them.

I also have bad news. None of them will work until you do something incredibly difficult. I'm going to ask it of you now, but it might be something that takes weeks, months, or even years to achieve. It certainly did for me.

You have to accept that the past is gone. Not just in a logical, literal sense, but in an emotional sense, too. No matter how well these strategies work for you and how hard you work, you will never feel exactly the way you once did. Even if you could go back in time and re-experience the same moments in the same body, they would feel different to you because you are no longer the same person who had those experiences the first time they happened. That doesn't mean your life won't be just as good, or even better in some ways, but it will be different. There's no way around that.

Although you can never re-experience the precious moments from your past, you can have experiences in the present that are just as meaningful to you in the future as the past is to you in the present. It's so easy to misunderstand what made the past feel the way it did to you. It wasn't the people, the places, the era, the activities, the music, or whatever else you think it was; it was your state of mind. We need to replicate that internal state of mind rather than the external elements of those moments if we want to make more of them.

Trying to relive or re-create your past is an exercise in futility. Cherish those special, sacred memories forever, but do not try to make more just like them because you'll never be able to. That isn't as tragic as it might sound. Part of what makes those memories so special is knowing that they were unique and time limited. To quote Brad Pitt as Achilles in the movie *Troy*: "Everything is more beautiful because we're doomed. You will never be lovelier than you are now. We will never be here again."

You need to be willing to have new, different experiences and try your best not to compare them to your past. If you compare them, they will never measure up because you're comparing an actual, warts-and-all present-moment experience to a glitchy VHS memory that's been extensively glazed over with seven layers of nostalgia. That's always going to result in a losing battle for the here and now.

The only way you'll ever have a moment in the present that means as much to you as the moments from your past is if you stop comparing the present to the past.

Doing It Like It's the Last Time

Perhaps the simplest technique, yet sometimes the most effective, is to ask yourself: *How would I engage with this activity if I knew I would never get to do it again?* It's very rare that we knowingly do something for the last time. Most endings slip into our lives under cover of night and don't reveal themselves until years later when it's far too late to appreciate what we've lost.

I almost certainly will not realize when I'm reading a book to my daughter or playing hide-and-seek with my son for the last time. It's so automatic for me to view these moments as mundane because, at this phase of my life, they are common experiences. But they won't be forever. Someday they will stop, and I won't know that those phases of my life are over until I start to miss them. Something else will replace them, and what comes next may objectively be even better, but there will still be grief when I realize that these experiences only exist in my memories.

There are parts of the life you have right now that are incredibly precious to you and that you will miss tremendously when they're gone. This trick can help you identify them and try your best to appreciate them before that moment comes.

I didn't know that my last time on the farm was my last time on the farm. I didn't intend for it to be. Had I known, I'd like to think that I would have handled it very differently. There will always be grief when something ends, and the grief can be crippling when we lose something we truly loved. There's no way to prevent this. It's simply the inherent price tag of having things in our lives that matter. However, we can minimize the magnifying impact that regret has on grief by keeping the temporary and precious nature of things within our conscious awareness.

I recommend using this technique sparingly. Maintaining a constant awareness of the temporary nature of everything in your life could easily lead to obsession, perfectionism, and paranoia. It can also be horribly depressing to remember that everything that you love will eventually end, even if what comes next is just as good, if not better. The ideal level of awareness is somewhere in between *This is something I'll always have* and *Every second of every day is precious and if I don't appreciate it I'm a horrible person.* Aim for the midpoint between these two extremes and adjust accordingly.

Remembering What It's Worth to You

It's difficult to appreciate things that we cannot attach some type of value or metric to. You know approximately how much your house and your car are worth, but for most of us, material possessions are not the most important part of our lives. Our relationships, experiences, feelings, and memories are often our most prized "possessions," but since they cannot be bought or sold, they don't necessarily make us feel "wealthy" the way we imagine tangible, material possessions would.

One of the best ways to appreciate something is to know its value, and one of the best ways to know the value is to estimate how much money it would take for you to part with it. Even if you never would or physically can't, a price tag gives us something measurable to associate with what we already have and helps us more fully appreciate it.

Consider something you have in your life right now that is incredibly precious or important to you. This could be anything that you personally find important: a person, a status, or an experience, to provide just a few examples.

How much would somebody have to pay you to take that thing away from you? Millions? Billions? Or maybe you simply can't put a price on it because you literally wouldn't trade it for anything material or tangible in this world?

Whatever your answer is, you currently possess something worth that much to you. I know it doesn't feel like it on a day-to-day basis, but that's just one of those annoying brain glitches we all have to deal with. Things that are normal do not feel special regardless of their actual value to us.

For example, I would not sell my wife for a billion dollars. Not only because selling humans is illegal and would land me in prison where I'd be unable to enjoy my wealth but also, and more importantly, because she is worth more than that to me. The cumulative positive impact she already has had on my life and will continue to have on my life is something I could never hope to purchase with any amount of money.

Because of this, I should feel happier and more content with my life every day that I'm married to her than I would if I had a billion dollars in the bank. If I don't feel that way on a daily basis, it's because I'm taking the wonders of my current life for granted, not because I don't have wonderful things currently in my life.

The same is true of you and what you already have. You are at least a millionaire, if not a billionaire. Your fortune is not liquid; you cannot cash in on it, and you never will. But you wouldn't want to anyway. You've already found at least one source of true wealth in this life; you just need to remember that you already have it.

If money isn't something you find yourself longing for, feel free to use another metric in its place. Shortly after my social media presence began to grow substantially, I was watching my young daughter splash around in the bathtub and found myself thinking about how incredible it would feel to have a billion followers. The influence, validation, and connection would be unreal. When I looked into my daughter's eyes, I impulsively said to her, "I wouldn't trade you for a billion followers." I needed a reminder that I already had something worth more to me than what I was longing for.

Imagine You Were the Only One

We tend to associate scarcity with value. Our lives contain so many wonderful experiences, people, statuses, and inventions that would have once been unfathomable to human society. One of my favorite ways to remind myself of the incredible value of what I already have is to pretend that I'm the only person who has it.

If you have children, how would it feel to be the only person on Earth who had the privilege of raising children? Can you imagine how special every moment of parenting would be if you were constantly aware that you and you alone were the one given this incredible gift? If that concept lands for you, why should the existence of other people's children lessen your appreciation of your own?

If you enjoy your career, how special would it feel to know you were the only person alive who got to do it? Ignore the pressure and the unreasonable demands that would come with this scenario if it were real (as a therapist, I would not actually want to have a caseload of roughly five hundred million people) and just focus on the emotional experience of it.

Or what about your home? If every other human being on Earth lived in tents or makeshift temporary shelters, and you were the only one with protection from the elements, central heating and air-conditioning, and consistent access to clean water, how easy would it be for you to see the incredible wonders and blessings present in your everyday life? Again, why should other people also having these things make them any less special or meaningful to you? The only thing standing in the way of your enjoyment and appreciation of the wonders of the present is your perspective.

Asking Your Butler to Do It

This technique works on two levels. It provides legitimate gratitude and appreciation for the wonderful things you have, but it also serves as comic relief. I've found that important concepts often slip past my defensive skepticism when they're hidden inside a Trojan horse of humor.

Nearly every one of us currently enjoys a quality of life that is dramatically better than that of the wealthiest kings hundreds of years ago. Sure, they had massive castles and armies of servants, but do you know what they didn't have? Toilets that flushed. Accurate climate control. Refrigerators. Electricity.

When you're struggling to appreciate the conveniences and luxuries of your life, remember that at one point you would have to either do all of these things yourself or hire someone to do them for you. On the days when I need to remember how good I have it, I pretend that I have an invisible butler named Jeeves who has to manually complete every task that inventions have automated. To provide some examples:

"Jeeves, allow the castle to reach a temperature of exactly sixty-five degrees Fahrenheit while I slumber in order to maximize the quality of my sleep. However, stoke the heart of the fireplace such that the castle temperature rises to exactly seventy degrees Fahrenheit before I awake, lest I grow chilly." (Programmable thermostat.)

"Jeeves, prepare the horses for the journey such that they do not struggle to pull the carriage despite the foul weather today. Have them run in circles for five to ten minutes prior to my departure so that they are ready to run the moment I enter the carriage. Also, rub a heated rock on my seat such that my backside will not be cold when I sit down." (Remote start.)

"Jeeves, light a fire in the cooking hearth and place upon it a bowl containing the portions of last night's dinner that I did not consume. Warm the food to a temperature that is warmer than this room but not as hot as the food was when it was first cooked, lest it become hard and chewy." (Microwave.)

"Jeeves, light three dozen candles throughout the house so that I continue to read and write long after the sun has set. I do not wish to be bound by the laws of nature tonight." (Light switches.)

I am not the least bit ashamed to admit that Jeeves has pulled me back from the brink of a foul mood on more than one occasion. It's just really hard to be upset when you have a butler.

Taking Inventory

One of the most common reasons that we take the wonderful things we have in life for granted is that we literally forget that we have them. Our minds are designed in a way that causes them to focus much more on what we don't have than what we do have, to value acquisition much more than retention. This leaves us chronically unsatisfied and disenchanted with what we have and filled with a longing to acquire more.

Imagine coming home one day to a pile of ashes where your home used to be. Everything you had is gone. All the things you took for granted, the possessions that never satisfied you, went up in smoke. The house itself, the one you often thought about selling or renovating, suddenly seems precious now that it's been burned to the ground. You have to start all over again from scratch. Your insurance adjustor asks you to make a list of everything that was lost.

Make that list today. Start from memory and write down everything you already have that's precious to you. Search your mind for everything you've coveted and acquired. Think of your keepsakes, your hobbies, and your luxuries.

Once you can't think of anything else, walk around your house and add to the list. Take your time with this process, fully exploring every room in your house and taking notice of everything you find that feels important to you. Make a full, complete inventory of everything you already have that matters to you.

Once that list is complete, take some time to look it over. Notice how it feels inside to consider all of the wonderful treasures you already have. Some you worked hard for, pulling extra hours or working side jobs to make a little extra so you could afford them. Some are precious gifts from people still in your life and some from those who are gone. You may even have things you yourself have built with just your body and your wits.

I hope you find the list at least a little bit impressive. You've worked hard for everything you have, and you deserve to feel good about that.

My fifth lesson to you is this: Remember the most precious parts of your life, no matter how common or mundane they may seem. Whether you realize it or not, you're an emotional billionaire with many precious things in life that nobody else has. Your challenge is to recognize and appreciate these things before you lose them. You can't trust your mind to automatically orient itself towards what matters to you; you have to initiate and consistently maintain this process manually or you risk taking incredibly precious things for granted. If you never forget what is special about today, you will finally stop chasing the past and start appreciating the present.

Truth Six

Keep the Water Flowing

The Story

The River

The water was so clean it sparkled in the sun. Shallow current rushed over blue-gray rocks of varying sizes before plunging into pools so deep I couldn't see to the bottom. The endless sound of flowing water created a soothing soundtrack I could never tire of hearing, especially when it was accompanied by the songs of frogs, crickets, and locusts. The canopy of green trees overhead provided much-needed shade on hot summer days.

Most of my waterfront life was spent around lakes, but the river was no less beautiful. It was just different. Schools of hundreds, if not thousands, of minnows darted through the shallows. The deeper pools held bigger fish that snuck to the surface anytime an unfortunate bug crash-landed into the water, assuming the frogs lurking on shore didn't get to it first. Turtles sunned themselves on logs while ducks and geese floated leisurely downstream with the current, snacking on nymphs and larvae along the way. Occasionally the peace would be broken by the jarring sound of a deer crashing through the water.

The Greek philosopher Heraclitus once stated, "No man ever steps in the same river twice, for it's not the same river and he's not the same man." The tremendous insight of this observation might be lost on someone who has never lived on the river, but he couldn't be more right. Just like our lives themselves, the river truly does change with every passing moment.

Because of the constant flow of water, things are always moving beneath the surface. Large or small, almost nothing stays in one spot for too long. Sand, silt, and pebbles are kicked up constantly, changing the depth of every point along the river bottom ever so slightly. Old fishing holes become shallow and barren over time, but new ones are being created constantly. Logs we used to sit on are washed downstream, while new shelters and places of respite come from upstream. It's a story with a new chapter every day, just like us.

Each season presents a different version of the river. No trace of life can be seen in the water just after the snow melts. It's a beautiful but empty display, like an ornate frame without a painting inside. Fish slowly move in from larger rivers throughout the spring, heading farther upstream to escape predators and looking for prey of their own, like the tadpoles and bugs that start to appear around this time. Summer brings spawning, fish beds, eggs, and thousands of minnows and fry. In autumn, the surviving babies enter their adolescence and prepare to move back into deeper water for the winter to avoid freezing.

I'm not sure whether it ended up there intentionally or by accident, but there was a massive, hollow concrete cylinder in the shallows just a couple of blocks from our home. It must have been eight feet long, easily large enough for a person to lie on. Some days the only way I could find any sense of peace or solace was to escape society, go down to the river, lie down on the cylinder, and close my eyes for a while. The fish and the animals would be my only companions. I'd focus all my attention on the sound of the water, the warmth of the sun on my face, and the wind blowing through the trees and, for a moment, I would find peace. At least until a deer would crash through the water and give me a panic attack.

I'm thankful that nobody ever discovered me at my little nature retreat. It would have made for quite a sight. Between my pale skin, long black hair, numerous piercings, and ripped baggy black clothes, I looked like somebody you'd expect to see at a metal concert, not stumble across performing a nature meditation in the middle of an idyllic stream.

Despite being in the middle of a city and receiving constant runoff from yards and roads, the main channel of the river always looked relatively clean. Sure, there were occasional tires and pipes and pieces of people's landscaping, but the water itself remained beautiful. The constant flow of the current carried anything that wasn't solidly part of the river, like trash or small branches, rapidly downstream.

I loved almost every inch of that river. I loved the rapid shallows. I loved the deep pools where the larger fish lurked. I loved the frogs and the turtles. I loved the little crawdads hiding under the rocks. I even loved the tires. The only part I didn't love was the backwater. We avoided that area at all costs after our first encounter with it.

From a distance it looked intriguing, a tiny pond just barely connected to the main channel by a thin stream of water. The closer we got, the more foreboding it appeared. The water was filthy, a dark brown stew bubbling ominously like a witch's cauldron. Plastic bags and wrappers lined the outer edge of the water. We had no idea how deep it was, so we did what young boys without a fully developed sense of self-preservation typically do: ignored the insistent tapping of fear on our shoulders and pushed ignorantly forward.

My brother went first. He took two steps into the water and proudly declared it wasn't very deep, barely up to his knees. As he was proclaiming this, the water appeared to be slowly rising around his legs. I realized it before him, but I thought he was pranking me somehow as he did from time to time. When we locked eyes, I saw the panic before he spoke it: He was sinking into the ground!

I rushed forward, grabbed his wrists, and pulled. Nothing. I pulled again. Nothing. Panicking, I grabbed on even tighter and launched myself backward in a sort of awkward horizontal jump. This time he came flying with me, collapsing into a heap on top of me.

We looked back at the water he came from in disbelief. A pair of rubber cylinders rose prominently from where he had been standing a moment ago.

I hadn't pulled him out of the mud. I had pulled him out of his boots, which the mud had retained a chokehold on. In just a few seconds he had sunk several inches into the river bottom, which had immediately closed back up around his soles. Even without his body weight in them, retrieving his boots from the mud required substantial effort.

I'm sure he would have stopped sinking eventually, but the sudden and unexpected brush with apparent danger in such an idyllic place was jarring to both of us. We noticed an odd aroma lingering in the air around his "rescue spot," an unpleasant scent that fell somewhere between "gas leak" and "sewage." Between the panic and the smell, we decided to be done exploring for the day.

The backwaters of rivers and streams have no current, nothing to create flow or movement. The water inside of them stagnates, not moving in any particular direction but sitting there lifelessly. This creates a completely different ecosystem from everything surrounding it.

Muck and sludge build up in the backwater with nothing forcing them to move downstream. The water contains high levels of carbon monoxide and swamp gases, the sources of the mystery aroma that permeated the air after my brother sank into the mud. Algae covers the surface of the water before dying in late fall and descending to the bottom of the river to rot, causing the backwater to look less like part of a beautiful stream and more like a dirty puddle full of rancid chocolate milk.

Garbage and debris that end up in the river normally float downstream, but anything that ends up in the backwater stays there. It's a veritable magnet for trash. Unlike the rest of the river, the backwater doesn't change every day. In fact, it almost never changes, other than in response to major weather events like floods. In backwaters, my brother and I have found beer cans and containers sporting designs that haven't been printed in twenty years. It's yet another space lost in time, but not in a good way.

Some types of animals can do very well for themselves in the backwater. Frogs, turtles, and snakes are well adapted to the stagnant conditions and often thrive in them. The smell of the stagnant water attracts plentiful bugs, making it a food hot spot for any resident insectivores. Raccoons sometimes find a treasure trove of oysters trapped in the stillness.

But most of the animals living in and around the river, particularly the fish, avoid the backwater at all costs. The dirty, gaseous water isn't oxygenated enough for most of them, and the garbage and plastic bags are traps, if not tombs, for anything that swims.

Everything disgusting, unpleasant, or scary about the backwater is a direct result of the lack of flow and current. The river needs to keep itself moving to stay clean and healthy. People's garbage ends up in it through negligence. Fish and animals die, and their carcasses float down to the bottom. Plants and weeds turn to muck and sludge each winter. All of this debris must be cleansed from the main channel and taken farther downstream or broken into tiny particles by the force of the water, or else they quickly build up into something very problematic. Long periods of stagnation make things disgusting, dangerous, and frankly, a little depressing.

The Lesson

Stuck in the Mud

Despite the tremendous challenges I've already told you about in these chapters, some of the hardest periods of my life have been the times when nothing really happened. Isolation can be miserable. Failure is painful. Grief is dreadful. But stagnation can be just as awful in its own way.

Even when life is relatively good, excessive sameness and repetition seem to build up emotional sludge and muck inside of me that suddenly have nowhere to go. My desire to continue to put forth the considerable effort necessary to sustain my existence slowly slips away without a constant outlet, an inner flow to keep the dark thoughts and feelings moving and preventing them from attaching themselves permanently to anything inside of me. Without something to move towards, some sense of meaning and purpose, the lack of a major acute problem never seems to be enough to keep me content.

During the stagnant periods of life, it often feels like I take care of myself mainly to go to work. I go to work so that I have an income. I need an income so that I can have the resources to take care of myself and my family. A family that, one hundred years from now, will have mostly, if not entirely, forgotten me. Sometimes I feel like a surge protector plugged into itself or an Ouroboros eating its own tail. Every reason to exist and thrive seems cyclical and self-referential. It doesn't take much to convince me that none of it really matters.

I know that some people find tremendous freedom and relief in the idea that our lives aren't objectively very important. Unfortunately for me, I am not one of those people. The idea that all of this striving and toiling functionally adds up to absolutely nothing just makes me want to rage quit the game. If there's no purpose, I don't want to play.

Purpose is an incredibly difficult thing to find. Like sleep, it cannot be forced or simply consciously decided upon. It's also tremendously challenging to hold on to even when you do find it because, as we've already discussed, we get used to whatever we have, and the emotions associated with having it begin to fade.

Finding a partner gave me purpose for a while. Feeling that unmatched sense of connection and shared ambition was my reason for waking up, my motivation for studying and going to the gym, the North Star guiding me towards a healthier, better version of myself. Just knowing that she existed and thought about me regularly was all I needed to face whatever demons the world saw fit to send my way on any given day. We're still together, and I love her even more than I did then, but my stupid brain adapted to her presence in my life and eventually started taking her for granted. I can, and do, consciously remind myself of how wonderful she is and how lucky I am to have her, but it isn't a constant feeling in the forefront of my mind as it once was.

When we had a child, that spark was reignited by a different kind of love. Now there was someone depending on me who legitimately could not take care of himself, someone who needed me in an even more literal, visceral way. Just knowing that he existed in this world filled me with a sense of meaning even when I wasn't consciously thinking of him. Despite the challenges and frustrations that inherently come with having a newborn (especially one like ours who resisted sleep with every fiber of his being and seemed to hate going anywhere—no idea where that came from), I once again felt like I had a reason to be alive, a valid justification to keep going. This feeling lasted the better part of two years, but then it, too, began to fade into the background of my mind, except for the occasional special moments that bring it to the forefront again.

Our second child had a complicated entry into this world and has a lifelong disability of unknown severity. When she wasn't walking or talking at age two, we consulted with specialists. I'll never forget the day I came home from work and her care worker had her in "walking wings" to support her in taking her first steps. The reality of our situation fully hit me in that moment: We had a child with significant challenges who was going to need a lot of support. Of course I was scared and concerned, but I also felt more certain than ever that I had a reason to be here. As of this writing she is eight years old and doing well, which is wonderful, but the spark of urgency I felt when I fully realized and accepted the fact that I was a special needs parent has become more of a background process at this point, as everything eventually seems to.

This process was repeated time and time again with graduations, promotions, starting businesses, creating social media content, mentoring young professionals, moving into new houses, and writing books. Each of them filled me with drive, ambition, and purpose for a while, but none of them lasted forever. Eventually every one of them fizzled out and plunged me back into the cold, dark, lonely void of my mind.

I've come to believe that purpose is more of a feeling than a status, and like all feelings, it comes and goes, and it cannot be maintained indefinitely by anything in this world. You can have it—which I believe we all do at all times—yet not feel it at all. When we engage in emotional reasoning and believe that our feelings are an accurate reflection of reality—which they often aren't—we mistake our lack of a felt sense of purpose for an objective lack of purpose, and we feel a growing sense of frustration and despair until something sparks the feeling again.

Some of this constant devaluation of the wonders and blessings of life stems from complacency. As we've already discussed in other chapters of this book, fighting back against the mental processes that cause us to feel like our lives and the things in them aren't all that special is something we should strive to do every day. However, some of this mental adaptation is unavoidable no matter how hard we fight. Our minds are simply not designed to experience long-term satisfaction from what this life has to offer.

At the risk of mixing metaphors, I've found that, at least for me, the feeling of a sense of purpose is less like a possession that you can acquire and keep and more like a fire that has to constantly be fed with different types of wood. The flames of ambition inside of me quickly adapt to whatever fuel source was last used to kindle them, and they develop the unfortunate ability to burn through the same type of wood at incredible speed. I have to regularly feed the fire a new type of wood to keep it burning. Fortunately, there are many types of wood in this world.

It's often said in the field of professional mental health that a constant need to stay busy is a toxic trait, an avoidance strategy to dodge your darkest feelings rather than coping with them or simply accepting them. I strongly disagree. In fact, I view this perspective as one that originates from a person who does not fully and intimately understand the darkness that can live inside of the human mind, which is incredibly disappointing coming from a fellow mental health professional. I am not running from my pain. I'm just trying to maintain the upper hand in a battle that I can never truly win.

The darkness that lives inside of me cannot be defeated, only subdued and temporarily restrained. There is no move that I can make to win this battle permanently, no single decision I can make that will put a final, conclusive end to the war inside of me. The best that I can do is win as many individual days as possible. I accepted this a long time ago: that I will go to my grave still at war with my inner nemesis.

Like the river, I believe that we need to have some amount of current and flow to our lives. Even those among us who seem to have everything from the outside looking in still experience some degree of constant pain, frustration, resentment, and rejection. Our minds seem to hold on to unpleasant experiences much more readily than pleasant ones, turning us into organic damage collectors of sorts. Novelty, challenge, and excitement create the current that washes these experiences downstream and, eventually, out of our systems entirely.

Many of the darkest chapters of my life have mercifully ended when a new passion or pursuit has shown up to yank me out of the mud. Having something to move towards creates a sense of flow or current in my life that breaks up everything that builds up inside me during stagnant periods of life.

My theory is that we tend to move on from the pain of our past when enough changes have taken place between the then and the now, and the memories associated with the pain almost feel like they happened to a different person. When we go for years without growth or change, we feel like the same person the entire time. Major evolutions in our lives serve as demarcation points for the passage of time.

The version of me that experienced the worst this life has had to offer feels like a character from a book or a movie now because he is so very different from the person I am today. This dulls the pain of those memories, which is the only reason I can speak or write about them.

Some of the pursuits that have helped move me forward have been big, obvious things: a major step up in status and responsibility at work or school, an exciting new relationship, a sudden surge of desire to take care of my body with diet and exercise, or an unexpected sense of a spiritual connection, to share a few examples.

But not all of them have had major objective significance in my life. The little things can help just as much. Spontaneously discovering an interest in personal fragrance (what ignorant fragrance newbies would call "cologne") helped pull me out of one of the deepest depressions of my adult life. Understanding how to properly use power tools and complete home repairs assisted me in recovering from the grief of losing my grandmother. Discovering the wonders of smoking meat over smoldering wood may well have been the only reason I was able to survive the incredible grind of my graduate education.

I recognize that, individually, some of these things may seem frivolous or even a bit silly. Taken on their own, they don't represent much more than a tiny drop in the black hole of a bucket of pessimism and hopelessness. Yet in my experience, enough tiny drops can fill such a bucket, at least for a while.

The Application

Never Stagnate

There is a constant push and pull that we have to fight against: It isn't healthy for human beings to stagnate, but it isn't natural for us to constantly grow, change, and improve. We have an inner drive for homeostasis (wanting everything to stay the same because it feels safer), which conflicts with an inner need for progression, creating yet another war within. Too much change creates a raging river inside that sweeps away everything indiscriminately, but too little creates a murky backwater where nothing really happens.

We need some tangible sense of forward movement in our lives to avoid excess buildup of emotional muck, sludge, and trash. Our existence in this world creates an accumulation of pain and damage, much of which does not resolve automatically. Without having something novel and interesting to renew our minds and wash away the burdens of each day, we tend to reflect and ruminate on the pain of our past and the stress and uncertainty of our future.

Being stable and healthy is necessary, but not sufficient, for us to live fully satisfactory lives. Our minds will adapt to whatever we have and, before long, will begin to ask a question that can be very difficult to answer: *Now what?* Once we finally build the firm foundation we've been working on for so long, we suddenly realize that we forgot to plan what to place on top of it.

Sometimes the growth and challenges we need are built into our lives, and we don't need to do anything "extra" to create them. Changes that are forced upon us usually don't feel great at first, but sometimes they provide the exact growth-inducing stimulation that we need for the chapter of life that we're in. It's important that we try not to instantly judge change as "bad" but work on accepting that it is "uncomfortable," though uncomfortable doesn't inherently mean bad. Uncomfortable simply means "unfamiliar," and unfamiliar can be good.

However, we cannot assume that the inherent structure of our lives will provide us with everything we need. Many periods of life will be defined by the stability we worked so hard to create. After a lengthy period of security and stagnation, we're likely to find ourselves craving something new and exciting. During these times, we have to manually create the flow of progression that we need to stay healthy.

There are many ways we can do this. I'm going to share with you the main categories of additions to my life that have kept me moving as well as some specific examples within each category. Of course, these are not anywhere close to being comprehensive lists, just a few basic ideas to turn to when you feel stuck.

Hobbies

Sometimes just finding something in this world that you love to do is all that you need for a while. Hobbies can serve as a simple, easily accessible source of novelty and stimulation. The introduction of a new, lighthearted leisure activity (or a long-forgotten source of joy from earlier in life) can be exactly what we need to break free from a stagnant period of life.

For some of us, hobbies tend to fall by the wayside as we enter adulthood. We often feel pressured to remove anything from our lives that doesn't produce something of external value like income or social status. For others, hobbies take over our lives and become an obligation or an obsession rather than a source of occasional stress-free joy. If we can avoid both extreme ends of the spectrum and keep hobbies in the middle where they belong, as a fun addition to life that counteracts the constant stress and pressure of existence, they can do wonders for our mental health. Listed below are some of the hobbies that helped me and those I've worked with professionally regain much-needed current and motion in their lives.

- Board games
- Camping
- Card games
- Collecting
- Fishing
- Geocaching
- Hair/makeup
- Hiking
- Hunting
- Puzzles
- Rock tumbling/polishing
- Style/fashion
- Video games
- Watching sports

Skills

Most of my life has been marked by feelings of inferiority and insecurity. For a long time, I coped with these feelings by avoiding the activities and situations associated with anything I didn't feel like I was very good at. The longer I avoided, the stronger the feelings of inferiority and insecurity became. Eventually, my life felt like a high-stakes game of hide-and-seek where I desperately tried to conceal anything that I was secretly terrible at while putting my relatively few talents and skills in the forefront of my observable existence.

Deciding to finally face my insecurities and the (many) areas of life where I simply wasn't very skillful or talented has been incredibly rewarding. The more skills you have, the more confident you feel. I know that's not exactly a groundbreaking idea, but it's incredibly easy to underestimate the impact of growing your skill set. If you feel reasonably competent in most situations you're likely to encounter, so much of your general anxiety will simply melt away.

Facing your fears head-on and forcing yourself to develop in the areas you frequently find yourself avoiding can be a complete game changer for what it feels like to exist in this world. The more things you're good at, the more you enjoy life and the more easily you experience a sense of purpose. Below are some of the skills I've seen, or experienced, that can significantly move a person forward.

- Auto repair
- Baking
- Calligraphy
- Cooking
- Dancing
- Financial investments

- Gardening
- Home repair
- Horseback riding
- Landscaping
- Learning a new language
- Organizing/decluttering
- Origami
- Photography
- Playing a sport
- Raising animals
- Restoring antique furniture
- Singing
- Video editing
- Weight training

Knowledge

Learning doesn't always have to serve a practical purpose. Increasing your knowledge base about a topic that interests you for no reason beyond curiosity and a love of learning itself is a valuable endeavor. It's also a functionally limitless pursuit as you will never know everything about anything, so finding something in this world that fascinates your natural intellectual desire is like a gift that you get to open again and again.

Simply knowing more about the world around you, and how things came to be the way that they are, can increase your sense of connection to life and humanity. You might find yourself interested in a broad topic (such as history in general) or a very specific subgenre of your chosen topic (such as World War II history). Follow your organic interests and dive deeper into anything that excites you and stimulates your mind. Below are just a few broad ideas to get you started.

- Astronomy
- History
- Mechanics
- Nature
- Nutrition
- Philosophy
- Politics
- Psychology (not that I'm biased)

Creativity

If it feels like something is stuck inside of you and longing to be released, which it often does during stagnant periods of life, consider creative expression as a potential outlet. There is something uniquely special and rewarding about taking something that only exists inside of you and offering it to the world. I firmly believe that we all have something to offer, even if your early experiences in life taught you otherwise. For what it's worth, mine did, too.

If your creative expression is something you show to others, try not to get discouraged if people don't appreciate it at first. The main purpose of your creative expression is simply to get unstuck from stagnant periods of life, not to make you famous or develop into a side hustle. If other people happen to appreciate what you do, that's simply a wonderful but optional bonus. This is ultimately just to allow you to take something inside of you and put it out there for the world to see. Below are some general ideas for creative expression.

- Blogging
- Coloring
- Creating social media content
- Drawing
- Knitting/crocheting
- Metalworking
- Painting
- Playing an instrument
- Pottery
- Video game design
- Woodworking
- Writing fiction
- Writing music
- Writing nonfiction
- Writing poetry

Spirituality

This is not a religious book, but I am a religious person. I'm not ready to attempt to guide anyone other than myself and my family in any particular spiritual direction, but I will go so far as to say that for people with brains like ours, minds that are so easily prone to feelings of nihilism and worthlessness, not having any sense of religion or spirituality can be incredibly dangerous. I spent most of my life believing that I was a hollow, empty, organic shell lacking soul or purpose. Finding a set of spiritual beliefs that aligned with my experiences in this world was the turning point for me in this struggle, the missing piece I'd been searching for since I was young and lost.

There is nothing quite like the feeling of connecting with something bigger, older, and more powerful than yourself. That being said, I understand that faith is much like purpose itself in that it isn't something you can simply decide to have. I spent most of my life without it, and while I don't claim to know the exact formula for finding it, I do know that you're much more likely to find something when you're actively looking for it than when you're hoping for it to spontaneously appear in your life. Here are some ways I found it for myself:

- Reading religious texts
- Reading books about religion
- Attending religious services
- Joining study/discussion groups
- Prayer
- Listening to podcasts about religion
- Watching YouTube videos about religion

❦ ❦ ❦

Whenever you feel stagnant in life, please consider referencing this chapter for ideas on how to get unstuck. Just try a few things and see what sparks your interest. Try not to worry so much about the big picture here, and just focus on finding something that makes you want to wake up in the morning.

My sixth lesson for you is this: Never allow the natural current of your life to stagnate for too long. Just like the river, the trash and sludge and muck of life tend to build up within us if there isn't enough inner movement to keep it all from getting stuck. The longer we live, the more painful memories and experiences we acquire. We require a consistent flow of novel thoughts and feelings inside of ourselves to break up these experiences and move them downstream, keeping our main channels clean. Try to keep at least one new, interesting thing happening in your life as often as possible to avoid turning into an emotional backwater of misery and regret.

Conclusion

Patterns

I want to spend the remainder of this book discussing a pair of patterns I've observed in my life that, while critical, don't require their own chapter. Understanding and applying these brief principles will increase the effectiveness of all the lessons I've shared with you, so please take your time with them.

Winning Strategies Change Over Time

So many of the sticking points we face in our respective journeys are a direct result of applying a solution that worked for a problem we faced in the past to a problem in the present that is just different enough to require a new strategy. If we wish to successfully overcome the next barrier life throws at us, subtle changes in the challenges that we face necessitate corresponding changes in our solutions.

Improvement often happens through a series of progressions and plateaus. We have periods of upward trajectories, when growth and improvement occur, and periods of flat trajectories, when we can't seem to figure out how to move forward. The flat trajectories often represent periods of constraint when we need to develop a new set of strategies to break down that next wall, like reaching the next level of a video game and realizing the new enemies have different attack patterns that we don't understand yet.

It's important to realize that this pattern of growth and stagnation is incredibly normal, or else you might become discouraged. My natural, knee-jerk reaction to hitting that next wall tends to be overly negative, often something along the lines of *I guess I'm not as good as I thought I was* or *See, I knew I couldn't really do this.* However, I've been through this cycle enough times to know that after I throw my little inner temper tantrum and look at the situation with less reactionary emotion and more mental objectivity, I'll eventually identify a solution. Ironically, the biggest barriers to moving forward are usually the wall within me, made up of my feelings of frustration and despair, and my insistence that what has worked before must work again.

The first time you read this book (because you're going to read it more than once, right?), there might be a certain chapter that stands out to you above the others. This is likely going to be the chapter with the greatest current applicability to your situation, the one written about a phase of my life that closely mimics yours. Hopefully you use the lessons I learned from my own struggles and progress beyond those internal barriers, but you'll likely reach a point where continuing to use the techniques from that chapter produces little benefit for you.

This doesn't mean that those strategies have stopped working or that you're doing them incorrectly—quite the opposite. It most likely means that you've used them effectively for a long time, have mostly overcome the challenges that they can help with, and now need to focus on something else to pass the next level. You may find that upon rereading the book a different chapter stands out to you, and the lessons from that chapter are exactly what you need to leap over the next hurdle.

It can be extremely difficult to accept that the strategies that served you so well in one chapter of life can be unhelpful—even a liability—in the next chapter, but it's a pattern I've experienced and observed on countless occasions.

The difference between dating success and long-term relational success is a good example of the need for shifting and evolving emotional strategies. In the early stages of a dating relationship, we all engage in heavy impression management. We put what we believe are the best parts of ourselves on display for potential partners to see and keep the damage and the dysfunction that we all have hidden behind a curtain of intrigue. If you fill your dating profile with red flags and character flaws, and regale your dating partners with stories of failures and setbacks, you are unlikely to have many second dates.

However, if you've been in a committed romantic relationship with a partner for quite some time, they most likely want to eventually see what lies behind that curtain. They want to know the real one, the one that nobody else gets to see, the person behind the mask. If you're never able to drop your guard with someone who works very hard to present themselves as safe, supportive, and trustworthy to you, that person may eventually become frustrated and leave.

Every phase of your life will require something new from you, so be prepared for a never-ending process of shedding old skin and redefining what it means to be you. Try not to rigidly cling to the techniques and tools that worked so well for you in the past. Be grateful to them and don't forget them, but don't expect one effective strategy to carry you from your current spot to the finish line. More than anything else, this life requires adaptation.

Excessive Focus on the Past Will Leave You Stuck

This point may seem ironic or even a bit tone-deaf given that we are nearing the end of a book that is two-thirds about my own past, but I've shared my past with you for purely illustrative purposes, not because that's where my answers were found. I didn't identify the principles I've shared with you in this book by endlessly ruminating on the parts of my life that had already happened, but by focusing on the present and noticing that the patterns playing out mimic principles I had seen demonstrated in earlier chapters of my life.

Your past is not an actionable time frame. You have no agency over history. We tend to analyze and replay the worst moments of our respective pasts to look for solutions to our present challenges, but the past rarely holds such answers. More often than not, spending a lot of time thinking about events that have already happened, especially those that didn't go the way we wanted them to, just creates a lot of present feelings of guilt and shame, which are counterproductive and antagonistic to positive change and growth.

If you're driving on the highway and you suddenly find yourself with a flat tire, there's no real benefit to looking at where you were driving before the flat happened to try and figure out what punctured it. You will probably never find it, and even if you do, it won't change the problem you're facing in the present: You'll still have a flat tire, and you still won't be getting home until you either patch and inflate it, switch it for a spare, or call a tow truck. Focusing on fixing the flat and getting home is more important than focusing on how you got the flat.

Very rarely do we find the answers we're looking for in our own personal history. The web of events that causes you to experience unusually strong reactions to certain situations is almost impossible to unravel because it's very rarely the product of any single experience or relationship. We are a product of everything that has ever happened to us, and every day of our lives shapes and molds us to some degree. This is even true in the case of life-changing traumatic events. Those events cause fallout, and it is often the complex aftermath of how well (or poorly) we handled that fallout that alters the course of our lives, more so than the events themselves.

That being said, I have occasionally seen therapy clients have "the moment" where something from their past clicks with something from their present. They realize they became a workaholic the first day they had a B on a report card and their parents disapproved, or that they developed body-image struggles when their grandmother made an offhand comment about their size when they were twelve years old. Do you know what changes in their lives once they have these revelations?

Nothing.

They come back for therapy the following week as the same person with the same problems and a little more insight. They know what punctured the tire, but it's still just as flat.

Knowing why you have a problem does not make the problem disappear. I think this is the biggest misconception about human insight: that knowing why we act some certain way is not only necessary for change but a catalyst for change. It is neither. Knowledge, in and of itself, changes nothing. It is also unnecessary for change.

You can fight against your workaholic tendencies, without fully understanding why you have them, by changing and redirecting present thoughts and behaviors. You can challenge body image distortions without tracing their lineage; you just need to speak truth to them. You do not have to fully understand yourself to change yourself, which is good because none of us will ever fully understand why we are the way we are. It would be like trying to watch every video on YouTube. There's simply too much data to sift through, and more is being generated every second.

Try to minimize the amount of time you spend digging through the wreckage of your past. I know that it's easier said than done, but simply setting it as a goal and labeling it as a generally fruitless activity will help immensely. Insight is not completely worthless, but it is vastly overrated.

The End, for Now

Another "normal" day comes to a close for me as I say good night to my children and spend a little alone time with my wife before heading to bed myself. I need to make sure I'm well rested for what will certainly be a full week of helping people deal with their darkest struggles—struggles that are often very similar to those I've faced in the past.

It tends to be in the moments when I'm sitting with someone who is in the middle of a very dark chapter of their life that I realize just how much my own has changed. I thought I would always be the one being helped (or, more accurately, resisting the help that was offered), rather than a person who had anything of value to share with others. My bad days now are better than my good days once were. My floor is well above what used to be my ceiling.

I know beyond any doubt that the experience of existing in this world can feel incredibly different (and better!) from one chapter of life to the next, but I also know how difficult it is to create those changes if, like me, you're starting from a very low and a very dark place. If you want to radically change what you get out of this life, you need to make a corresponding radical change in what you put into this. This change will likely need to be comprehensive—an overhaul of mind, body, and spirit. It has been my goal to make such a change feel possible, by example, and give you a sense of where to start (or where to go next if you've already begun the process).

I sincerely hope that this brief glimpse into some of the most challenging periods of my life, and my methods for overcoming these challenges, provides you with some of the tools you need to do the same. More than anything, I hope you feel some sense of connection to me now that I've shared some of my most vulnerable thoughts and feelings with you. I know all too well how lonely and isolating this journey can be, and how it often appears that everyone in the world except for you is thriving with ease.

Many of those who look to be living their best lives are fighting battles very similar to yours, on the inside. If you met me in passing, you would never suspect that the words in this book came from somebody like me. Many people have felt the same way you feel, most just aren't willing to talk about it openly. We sacrifice so much potential for connection and support on the altar of impression management and projected strength.

If this book was helpful to you, I hope that you'll choose to connect with me on social media in some way. I regularly create content like what I've written here, so this is by no means the end of our time together. It could be just the start.

Goodbye for now, my friend.

Acknowledgments

This book could not have been made without the help and support of the following individuals. Thank you to . . .

My wife, Tracy Eilers, for being a responsible adult and managing our children and our home while I spent hundreds of hours in a quiet room typety-typing on my computer.

My children, Corey and Sadie Eilers, for occasionally telling me that they think it's cool that I write books.

My parents, Stan and Carol Eilers, for providing me with the experiences in this book, and for never giving up on me even when I gave them plenty of indications that it was probably the smart move.

My editors, Claire Schulz and Sarah Modlin, for being passionate about my work, helping me realize when I was nonsensically rambling, and finding every last misplaced indent, comma, and period (even the one I misplaced on purpose in this section.).

My publisher, BenBella Books, for making the process of creating a book from start to finish smoother than I imagined possible.

My literary agent, Giles Anderson, for being the only person who responded to my emails and helped me understand the publication process before I had a large following.

My social media manager, Tim Beehler, for helping me communicate my message more effectively.

My pastors, Steve Benton and Levi Anderson, for helping me understand the things that make no logical sense to my rigid intellectual brain.

My Lord and savior Jesus Christ, for literally everything.

About the Author

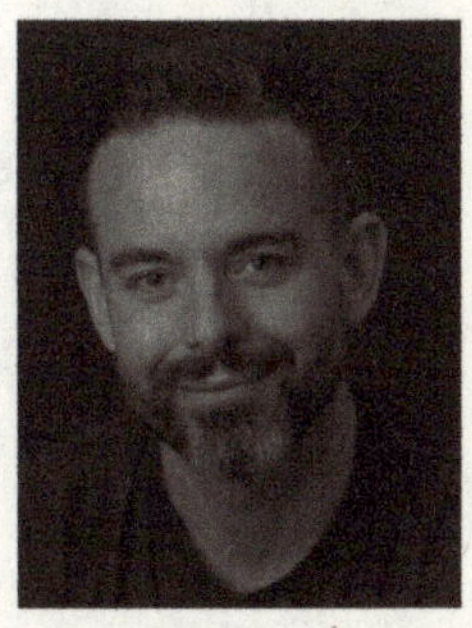

Scott Eilers, PsyD, LP, is a full-time board-certified clinical psychologist and the owner of the North Star Psychological Center. He has fifteen years of experience providing individual and group psychotherapy, mostly to individuals with relatively severe conditions such as bipolar disorder, severe depression, severe anxiety, post-traumatic stress disorder, borderline personality disorder, anorexia, and bulimia. He's also the author of *For When Everything Is Burning*, the host of the podcast *The Psychology of Depression and Anxiety*, and a regular content creator on YouTube, Instagram, and TikTok.